Enzymes: The Path to Perfect Health

Dr. Susan's Healthy Living
drsusanshealthyliving.com

Facebook.com/DrSusanRichards
drsusanshealthyliving@gmail.com
(650) 561-9978

Mention of specific companies or products in this book does not suggest endorsement by the author or publisher. Internet addresses and telephone numbers for resources provided in this book were accurate at the time it went to press.

ISBN 978-1511925235

Note

The information in this book is meant to complement the advice and guidance of your physician, not replace it. It is very important that any person who has medical problems be evaluated by a physician. If you are under the care of a physician, you should discuss any major changes in your regimen with him or her. Because this is a book and not a medical consultation, keep in mind that the information presented here may not apply in your particular case. In view of individual medical requirements, new research, and government regulations, it is the responsibility of the reader to validate health practices and treatments with a physician or health service.

Table of Contents

Part I:
Understanding Enzymes

1

How Digestive Enzymes Benefit Peak Performance and Health

Imagine a life in which you had the ability to eat a wide variety of foods from virtually any cuisine (a real benefit when traveling for business or pleasure) without any digestive discomfort. How would it feel to have tremendous levels of energy, the ability to work intensely without tiring, even for long periods of time when necessary, and still have plenty of energy to do your favorite activities like swimming hiking, golfing, painting, writing or cooking?

What if you could sit at the computer for hours on end without shoulder, neck or wrist pain, or even achiness and stiffness of your back? What if you could sit in the usually cramped accommodations of an airplane, for as long as fifteen to twenty hours, without feeling much stiffness or tiredness after the trip? How would it feel if you were able to recover rapidly from physical stresses and illness? Or, even better, what if you could enjoy great health and rarely get sick at all?

Abundant digestive enzyme production is the essential link for all of these positive qualities. Not only is digestive enzyme production crucial for processing and absorbing the food we eat, but it is a prerequisite for providing us with the energy and mental capacity to perform effectively in every area of our lives. Digestive enzymes help us perform well on the job and carry out our family responsibilities. They also enhance our ability to derive enjoyment from our activities and relationships as well as lead richly textured and pleasurable lives.

Extensive clinical experience and many research studies have shown that digestive enzymes also assist and speed up recovery from athletic and job related trauma and injury as well as dental procedures and surgery. Even more importantly, having abundant digestive enzymes plays a crucial role in protecting against and helping recover from a wide variety of inflammatory diseases, infections, auto-immune conditions, heart disease and even cancer. Enzymes literally create a protective shield within our bodies, helping to prevent the onset of many diseases. Yet, most people are unaware of how greatly digestive enzymes support our overall health and wellness.

Unfortunately, there are millions of individuals in the United States today who lack both the digestive firepower and the energy to perform to their own goals and expectations and live life to the fullest due to inadequate digestive enzyme production. Even if an individual does not possess a peak performer's digestive capability, the ability to restore this function is within everyone's grasp.

I have written this book to give you the essential resources to support your own digestive enzyme production as well as discussing the best enzyme supplements, their health benefits and how to use them. You will also learn about the chemistry of digestive enzymes, how they are produced within your body, and how diet, lifestyle, stress and aging affect your enzyme levels. Finally, I share with you valuable information about how to evaluate and test your own enzyme levels. At the end of this book, you will have all of the resources that you need for incredible health and wellness through supporting your own digestive enzyme levels.

The important benefits of digestive enzymes for peak performance and optimal health are listed in the following chart.

Benefits of Healthy Digestive-Enzyme Production

Peak-Performance Benefits

- Increased physical vitality and stamina (helps improve work productivity)
- Enhanced mental clarity and acuity
- Increased ability to get along with other people (permits enjoyment of extensive social and business entertaining)
- Hastened recovery from injury, and exertion (includes trauma and inflammation from athletic and repetitive-stress injuries; minor surgery; and dental procedures)

Health Benefits

- Optimizes digestion
- Improves absorption of nutrients and medications, thereby increasing their effectiveness
- Helps in the recovery from colds, flus, sinusitis, bronchitis, and allergies
- Lowers the risk of inflammatory diseases such as rheumatoid arthritis, colitis, endometriosis, prostatitis, interstitial cystitis, and thyroiditis
- Reduces menstrual cramping, helps to treat endometriosis and a variety of other female related conditions.
- Decreases the risk of and accelerates healing from heart disease, stroke, and blood clots
- Is used as a complementary therapy for the treatment of cancer

2

The Chemistry of Enzyme Production

Our bodies produce thousands of different enzymes, all catalyzing different chemical reactions that are crucial to health and survival. These reactions help regulate functions as diverse as the production of energy, digestion, the elimination of waste products, and the repair of cells. Thus, enzymes allow us to breathe, digest, grow, heal and perceive with our senses.

Enzymes affect chemical reactions in the following manner: An enzyme acts on another substance, called a substrate, grasping, holding, and binding the substrate with other molecules to help trigger a chemical reaction. Enzymes allow these reactions to proceed more efficiently, making it possible for them to occur with less expenditure of energy. Thus, an enzyme is a catalyst. Relative to the substances they are acting on, enzymes are present only in small amounts; moreover, enzymes are not changed by the biochemical process they help to initiate.

Because each enzyme has a unique shape that only fits with a certain substance, the various enzymes have very specific functions. For example, pancreatic enzymes, break down very specific types of food. Pancreatic protease enzymes digest only proteins, whereas pancreatic lipase is necessary for the proper digestion of fats, and pancreatic amylase works only on starch molecules.

The Essential Digestive Enzymes

The process of digestion is dependent on several dozen digestive enzymes that are produced by the body at different sites along the digestive tract: in the mouth, stomach, and small intestine. The activation of a digestive enzyme is regulated through changes in the pH (the relative acidity or alkalinity of the environment that the enzyme is operating in). Each part of the digestive tract has an optimal range of pH in which the digestive enzymes produced within that site can be activated and will also work most efficiently.

These enzymes break down the foods we consume into particles small enough to pass through the intestinal wall and then into the bloodstream. From the bloodstream, food particles are then absorbed into the cells where they are converted into usable energy.

The cells rely on a steady supply of nutrients from the blood to produce adenosine triphosphate (ATP), which is the main energy unit of the body. Our body uses ATP to fuel literally hundreds of thousands of chemical reactions. When the pancreas is producing adequate amounts of digestive enzymes, this process repeats itself meal after meal, providing the body with the nutrients needed to produce and sustain energy.

If digestive enzyme production is diminished, none of the food that we eat can be properly absorbed and assimilated by the body. This concept is often a surprise to many people, who assume that if they eat a lot of food, they'll be well nourished and healthy. However, a full plate doesn't always translate into a healthy body and a vital life, particularly if the body is unable to properly use the food we eat due to a lack of adequate digestive enzymes.

The Stages of Digestion

Ptyalin, a digestive enzyme found in saliva, begins starch and sugar digestion in the mouth. Sugar and starch break down relatively easily, compared with protein and fats, because of their simple structures. A molecule of table sugar is composed of just two molecules (glucose and fructose), and starch is composed of long chains of glucose connected together.

In comparison, proteins and fats have a more complex structure, and their digestion begins farther down in the digestive tract. Proteins are composed of various combinations of twenty-two amino acids. While the core structure of the amino acids is the same, they vary greatly in their chemical properties and in their effects on the body due to the varying side chains that branch off of every core chain.

There are also several different kinds of fats often found in the foods we eat. Much of our dietary intake of fat is in the form of triglycerides, which are composed of three fatty acids attached to a single molecule of glycerol (an organic alcohol). Phospho-lipids, an important component of cell membranes, differ from triglycerides in that they contain only a phosphatidylcholine molecule and two fatty acids attached to the glycerol (choline is a B vitamin). Cholesterol, a white, waxy, fatty material, is both found in our foods and produced within the body by the liver.

Most of the digestion occurring in the stomach relates to the breakdown of protein. Protein derived from meat and milk (casein) is particularly tough in texture and is either curd-like or fibrous. The digestion of protein in the stomach begins with the action of the enzyme pepsin. Pepsin is activated only in an acid environment. The necessary level of acidity is provided by the hydrochloric acid (HCl) secreted by the stomach, which allows digestion to proceed at an optimal pH of 1.8 to 3.5.

It is in the small intestine that the greatest amount of digestion of all types of foods occurs, whether carbohydrate, protein, or fat. The pancreas produces the digestive enzymes amylase, trypsin, and chymotrypsin, which further digest the molecules of protein and starch. Pancreatic lipases begin the digestion of fats. (These enzymes are discussed more fully later on in this chapter.)

The liver also secretes bile into the small intestines, which helps to emulsify or break up dietary fat. Water also plays an important role in the digestive process. Molecules of water in the gastrointestinal tract split large molecules of food into smaller, more absorbable units.

The Powerful Pancreatic Enzymes

Of all the digestive enzymes, pancreatic enzymes are among the most critical for the absorption of food and maintenance of good health. Pancreatic enzymes are also the most well researched of all the digestive enzymes, showing a wide variety of benefits essential for health and peak performance.

The pancreas is an organ that lies mostly under the stomach, except for one end, which is tucked into the curve of the upper intestine. Within the pancreas are special glands called acini that secrete digestive enzymes. These enzymes pass through a network of ducts that come together to form the main pancreatic duct and are then secreted into the small intestine.

Stored within the pancreas, the digestive enzymes are in an inactive form, preventing them from digesting the organ itself. Once secreted into the intestine, the stored form of trypsin is then activated — which, in turn, activates the other digestive enzymes.

Since pancreatic enzymes are activated only in an alkaline environment, pH plays an important role. The necessary alkalinity is attained through the secretion of bicarbonate-rich digestive juices, also produced by the pancreas. The pancreas secretes about 2.5 quarts of pancreatic juice each day.

The pancreas also contains the islets of Langerhans, which secrete important hormones including insulin, which regulates the level of sugar in the blood. Insulin is a protein that binds with sugar molecules and allows them to pass from the blood, across the cell membrane, and into the cell, where the sugar is used as the main source of energy for the cell. When insulin production is insufficient to clear sugar from the bloodstream, hyperglycemia or diabetes mellitus can result.

Pancreatic Enzymes and Digestion

Pancreatic digestive enzymes are capable of breaking down all types of food: carbohydrate, protein, and fat. The protein-digesting (proteolytic) pancreatic enzymes include trypsin, chymotrypsin, and carboxypeptidase. These enzymes can digest up to 300 g of protein per hour.

In the final stages of digestion, pancreatic and other enzymes break protein down into approximately twenty amino acids, which can then be readily absorbed into the bloodstream through the small intestine. These amino acids are then recombined into the various proteins needed to maintain both the structure and health of the body.

For example, proteins are an important structural component of tissues as diverse as hair, skin, blood, and bones. Important body chemicals such as antibodies, hormones, and all enzymes (not just digestive ones) are also composed of protein.

Pancreatic amylase digests starches, breaking them down into simple sugars. Starch-digesting enzymes can process up to 300 g of carbohydrate per hour. The pancreatic lipases help break down fats, oils, and cholesterol.

Fat-digesting enzymes can digest up to 175 g of fat per hour. Fats are first emulsified (split into tiny particles) within the small intestine by the action of bile salts from the gallbladder. Bile is a thick, bitter fluid secreted by the liver and stored in the gallbladder. It is composed of lecithin, cholesterol, bile salts, and bile pigments. Pancreatic lipase also continues the digestion of fat within the small intestine. Lipases break down large fat globules, but this action is much more effective when the fat has been emulsified first.

Animal studies suggest that the amount of pancreatic enzymes varies in relation to the composition of the diet. For example, a study published in the *American Journal of Physiology* found that laboratory animals produce a range of specific pancreatic digestive enzymes in response to eating certain foods.

The researchers fed rats a constant diet high in carbohydrates and observed an increased production of amylase. Rats on a high-protein diet produced higher levels of trypsin. Similarly, when you drink a glass of orange juice, your body produces amylase to digest the sugars and when you eat a shrimp cocktail, the pancreas produces proteolytic enzymes to break down the protein.

Research studies have confirmed that enzymes are absorbed from the intestinal tract into the circulation intact and still in active form. In one such study, reported in *Clinical Pharmacology and Therapeutics*, 21 healthy volunteers were given preparations of the enzymes bromelain and trypsin four times a day for four days. Researchers found that the blood levels of the enzymes rose with the administration of the supplemental enzymes.

Not only can supplemental digestive enzymes be absorbed into the circulation, but the body has a method to recycle and even reuse its own pancreatic enzymes. A study published in *Science* found that intact digestive-enzyme molecules, produced by the pancreas and excreted into the intestines, can be reabsorbed, stored within the body, and reused as needed.

This is an excellent example of the economy with which the body functions by reducing the demand on the pancreas to constantly produce new enzymes. Thus, the use of supplemental digestive enzymes, over time, will actually help to restore pancreatic function by reducing the workload of the pancreas.

Pancreatic Enzymes and Inflammation

A second important function of pancreatic digestive enzymes is to facilitate recovery from tissue damage or injury. All traumatic injuries are characterized by an inflammatory response. Similarly, internal injury to tissues due to such stressors as infectious bacteria, viruses, allergens, and toxins can cause inflammation.

Inflammation of an injured area is characterized by swelling, heat, stiffness, a reduced range of motion, and pain on weight bearing or use of the extremity or joint. No matter where the site of the injury, the physical manifestations are the same.

When an area of the body becomes inflamed, the blood vessels and capillaries in the injured area begin to dilate (expand), allowing fluids carrying the body's own healing substances to reach the area quickly. At the same time, the capillary walls become more permeable, and fluids force their way into the surrounding tissue, causing congestion. Very quickly more fluid and waste accumulate than the area can handle.

Helper cells seal off the damaged area, creating fibrin clots made of protein, to prevent the spread of bacteria and toxins to surrounding areas. The result is blockage of the blood and lymph vessels, leading to redness, swelling, heat, pain, and the formation of excess fluids in the tissue (edema).

The inflammatory process is controlled by numerous digestive enzymes, particularly proteolytic the body's own pancreatic protein-digesting enzymes, which eliminate debris at the injury site and initiate the repair of tissue. These enzymes also break up the fibrin, which is made of protein, so that it can be excreted.

Digestive enzymes keep the pathological process from spreading and considerably reduce the duration of the injury by speeding up the healing process. Thus, abundant production of digestive enzymes can greatly limit the severity and scope of inflammation diseases or external injuries.

Summary

Digestive enzymes, particularly pancreatic enzymes, are catalysts that break down the foods we consume into molecules that can pass through the intestinal wall and be absorbed by our cells. The cells then convert these molecules into energy.

Pancreatic enzymes are essential in the process of converting food into energy. A second important function of these enzymes is to break up inflammation caused by trauma, infections, allergens, and toxins and to initiate the repair of tissue; therefore, these enzymes help the body recover from injuries.

3

How Diet, the Aging Process, and Lifestyle Affect Digestive Enzyme Production

Many factors can affect digestive function, causing it to become less efficient. The production of pancreatic enzymes, in particular, may decline as a consequence of the normal aging process, poor dietary habits, excessive alcohol intake, and pancreatic and gall-bladder diseases. Each of these factors is discussed in detail in this section.

Diet and Eating Habits

The hard-to-digest standard American diet takes its toll on the digestive health of millions of individuals. As people adapt their eating habits to the reality of their busy lifestyles and schedules overloaded with work and family responsibilities, they are less likely to prepare the healthful meals, complete with enzyme-rich fresh fruits and vegetables, which are so necessary for good health.

In my clinical practice, I have seen thousands of patients who do not have the digestive health of their own parents and grandparents, who were raised in an era when synthetic and fast foods were much less prevalent. Meals were still prepared from scratch at home, and much of the food purchased, from grocery stores or roadside stands, was fresh from the farm.

The foods in the standard American diet, which is high in saturated fats, sugars, and animal protein, place a great demand on the pancreas. Hard-to-digest foods force the pancreas to secrete higher levels of digestive enzymes in order to break them down into small enough units that they can be absorbed across the small-intestinal wall and used as fuel by the cells.

Overworking the pancreas by eating high fat and sugary foods such as pizza, bacon, French fries, cheeseburgers, donuts, and chocolate cake can compromise pancreatic digestive-enzyme function and accelerate the aging of this organ. It is a health disaster in the making.

These foods are laden with saturated fats, red-meat protein, and sugar, which are commonly found in commercially prepared foods. People assume that if they are avoiding desserts and sweet baked goods such as cakes, pies, pastries, and cookies, they have eliminated sugar from their diet. But sugar and assorted sweeteners are also added to crackers, breakfast cereals, canned soups, ketchup, and pickles, among other dietary staples.

Digesting a meal high in fat, protein, and sugar requires a lot of energy, which is why people often feel so tired after a heavy meal. Symptoms of indigestion can be an early sign that the pancreas is stressed and unable to meet the demands being placed on it. Over time, an improper diet can increase the risk of diseases such as diabetes and pancreatitis.

Furthermore, the time pressures on many people, both in the business world and in family life, result in many meals being eaten hastily. People eat on the run, grabbing a quick bite at their desk or between appointments in their car. The millions of people who frequent fast-food outlets are testament to the hurried pace of modern life.

Janice is a patient that I worked with who was dealing with her constant anxiety and nervousness over the stresses of her life by drinking one diet soft drink after another throughout the day. She was clearly addicted to these unhealthy beverages. These drinks were leaving her feeling more tired and chronically in pain in her digestive tract because of the chemicals and acidity of these drinks. Her skin also looked very pasty and unhealthy.

I recommended that she switch to green tea or water with bitters and a touch of freshly squeezed limes or lemons. She began to notice a difference immediately and told me that her pain started to diminish and that she was feeling much better.

Between less than ideal meals, people are constantly snacking on foods and beverages that contain refined sugar, white flour, trans fatty acids (partially hydrogenated oils found in many cookies, crackers, and energy and breakfast bars), and caffeine.

Very little enzyme-rich, fresh food is consumed, creating stress on the pancreas, which leads to a reduction in its functional capability and premature aging. As a result, Americans in record numbers suffer from digestive complaints, low energy levels, and poor health. Look inside any supermarket or pharmacy and you will be astonished to see all the products being sold to treat digestive complaints.

A lifetime of unhealthy eating habits can accelerate the normal aging of the pancreas as well as the rest of the digestive tract. The following story illustrates this point. Some years ago I became acquainted with an affluent retired couple, Charles and Marie.

After spending many decades working hard at busy and successful careers, they embarked on a life of leisure and travel, taking four or five cruises a year. They both enjoyed the endless procession of meals on shipboard, starting with eggs Benedict and fresh-baked rolls and pastries for breakfast. This would be followed by lunches and dinners that included delicacies such as richly sauced red meat and seafood entrées, caviar and pâté, cheese trays and decadent desserts.

They both particularly enjoyed chocolate confections served at the end of the meals. Charles also frequently sampled the fine wines offered with the various courses. Finally, at tea time, there were trays of tarts and savory sandwiches to snack on.

However, Marie and Charles differed significantly in their ability to handle such rich fare. Marie is a true digestive peak performer. She has always been able to eat these meals aboard the cruise ships without suffering any digestive discomfort, and without the typical ten- to twenty-pound weight gain that many people incur on cruises.

Charles was not as fortunate. Although he endeavored to eat the same high-stress diet as his wife, his digestive function was not nearly as strong. He was constantly complaining about bloating, gas, and heartburn, which worsened over time.

After several years of feasting aboard cruise ships, he was diagnosed with gallstones and deteriorating liver health, with an elevation noted in his liver enzymes. After undergoing gallbladder surgery, Charles was warned by his physician to change his eating habits by adopting a low-fat, vegetarian-emphasis diet. But Charles ignored his doctor's warning and continued his life of feasting and leisure. Several years after his gallbladder surgery, unfortunately he was diagnosed with pancreatic cancer. He died within three months of diagnosis.

The story of Charles and Marie illustrates another important point: People who live together often have differing digestive capabilities. One of the partners in a relationship often has a much healthier digestive system than the other.

Often, the person with the "less sturdy" digestive capability will try to keep up with the stronger partner, with disastrous consequences. This is a difficult situation for many people because eating together provides enjoyment and is the social focus of many people's lives. For busy working couples, eating out or bringing home a takeout meal may be the only time they spend together.

Unfortunately, this can result in significant digestive stress for the person with a weaker digestive system and can eventually result in digestive problems as well as chronic fatigue and, even, serious illness.

If you lack the digestive stamina of your partner, always have dishes available that are easy for you to digest and do not put a strain on your digestive system.

Lifestyle and Health

Several other lifestyle factors besides diet and eating habits affect digestive-enzyme production, including caffeine, drugs, alcohol, and stress, as well as pancreatic disease, which may be caused by these factors. I discuss these various lifestyle factors in this section.

Stimulants

As the production of pancreatic enzymes begins to diminish, people often compensate for the decline in their energy by increasing their use of stimulants such as caffeine. Chemicals like caffeine hype the system, usually by over stimulating the adrenals and the nervous system.

However, these stimulants by themselves do not create or sustain long-term energy. Midlife and older people who are currently in the workforce often increase their use of stimulants to help them keep up with the demands of their jobs.

The National Coffee Association, based in New York, stated in their *Winter Coffee Highlights* report that people between the ages of fifty and fifty-nine consume the most coffee, followed by those aged forty to forty-nine, and then by those aged sixty to sixty-nine. Most people aged forty to fifty-nine are performing in the workplace even if they are not producing adequate amounts of energy.

Since digestive-enzyme production begins to decline around the age of forty, stimulants such as caffeine are used to generate the energy needed by midlife people to compete with younger workers, who still have relatively intact pancreatic function and a high level of energy.

Other stimulants like nicotine (found in cigarettes and drugs) may also be used by some individuals to bolster their level of energy. The use of stimulants to combat fatigue cannot sustain performance over time.

Dining While Traveling for Work

Millions of people travel regularly as part of their work. Business travel presents its own nutritional challenges. One major problem is that all business activities are concentrated into as short a time as possible. This often means that one is either entertaining or being entertained for breakfast, lunch, drinks, and dinner. Often, this means eating rich meals with wine or other alcoholic beverages.

In addition, when business people are away from home with nothing to do after work, they tend to reward themselves with rich meals on their expense account. If you are required to travel frequently for work and are having a hard time handling the stress of eating on the road, always travel with supplemental digestive enzymes. If you tend to be overly acidic, you will also want to travel with alkalinizing agents (see my book on pH and acid-alkaline balance for more information on this topic).

If your job requires you to travel extensively, either by car or plane, be sure to bring enzyme-rich snacks like raw sprouted seeds and legumes, which are crunchy and tasty. Other high-enzyme snacks include carrots and celery sticks, slices of green and red pepper, salads with fresh sprouts, or fresh fruit. These foods will help you maintain your energy much more effectively than the chips, candy bars, cola drinks, coffee, and fast foods that most people eat on the road or in airports.

Jeff and Helen's Stories

I would like to share with you the stories of two of my patients whose unhealthy dietary habits while working on the road caused an enormous amount of wear-and-tear on their bodies.

Jeff typifies the digestive decline that can occur when a person is required to travel frequently for business. A sales manager in his early forties, Jeff traveled between one-third and one-half of the time. His preferred dinner on the road consisted of steaks or chops accompanied by a baked potato filled with butter and sour cream, finished off with pie and ice cream.

Eventually, Jeff began to find that eating this customary meal triggered symptoms of heartburn, bloating, and abdominal cramps, and even more importantly, that his energy level was beginning to decline. Taking a red-eye flight for a breakfast meeting was becoming more difficult; energy would flag by midafternoon. It was also hard to maintain his energy and enthusiasm in business meetings that could last into the evening.

Although Jeff enjoyed his work, he began to consider finding a less stressful position with lower pay and less responsibility. Like Jeff, Helen's work required her to travel constantly. As a veteran flight attendant working on cross-country routes, she would eat the peanuts, pretzels, and cookies served to passengers as snack foods. The meals she ate on layovers were usually no more nutritious. She ate chocolate bars and drank caffeinated cola drinks each day for a quick energy boost and favored fast foods such as hamburgers and pizza.

By her mid-thirties, she was beginning to suffer from digestive symptoms such as bloating, gas, and indigestion as well as PMS-related fluid retention and mood swings. Moreover, she was finding it increasingly difficult to sustain the energy necessary to perform her job well.

Both Jeff and Helen contacted me for a nutritional consultation to relieve their symptoms. I worked with each of them to develop dietary programs that would enable them to continue their rigorous travel schedules and still maintain the level of energy necessary to perform their jobs.

Both Jeff and Helen began to order more wisely from restaurants, selecting more soups, salads, and vegetable side dishes. When Jeff felt the need for more protein, he ordered salmon or grilled chicken. Helen also began to carry her own snacks when flying, passing up the usual airline snacks in favor of fresh fruit, raw seeds and nuts, and rice crackers. Finally, they both began to take supplemental digestive enzymes with each meal.

Within several months, both Jeff and Helen began to experience higher levels of energy, and they found that they were once again able to handle the demands of their work.

Alcohol

The excessive use of alcohol stresses many vital organs of the body, including the liver, pancreas, and brain, causing inflammatory changes and destruction at the cellular level. Alcohol increases the risk of acute pancreatitis, a serious inflammatory condition that can become chronic and recurring if alcohol consumption is not curbed.

Because of the high rate of alcohol consumption throughout the world, the potential for disease of the pancreas is enormous. There are over 100 million regular drinkers in the United States alone. About 11 million Americans report heavy alcohol use, and more than half the population are social drinkers.

An even more alarming statistic is that for children and teenagers, alcohol consumption is on the rise. An estimated 5 percent of children ages twelve to seventeen consumed alcohol more than fifty days during the year. Individuals with poor pancreatic function should avoid alcohol entirely or only use it on special occasions (birthdays, holidays, and other celebrations). A serving should be limited to one 4 oz. portion of wine.

Fasting

When a person fasts, there is no food in the stomach and therefore no need to produce pancreatic digestive enzymes. In the fasting state, the pancreas becomes relatively inactive, and many functions slow, including enzyme production.

An animal research study on the effects of fasting, published in the *Proceedings of the Society for Experimental Biology and Medicine*, documented a decline in such basic biochemical processes as the synthesis of pancreatic DNA (deoxyribonucleic acid). Fasting can also cause the pancreas to lose its ability to secrete adequate levels of amylase, a starch-digesting enzyme, and when an individual eats again, the individual may have digestive problems if there is a high amount of starch in the meal. Symptoms include intestinal discomfort, excessive gas, and bloating.

Gas is produced when undigested and unabsorbed nutrients travel to the colon, where the resident bacteria ferment them, producing gas as a by-product. The most common gases produced by bacteria in the intestines are odorless: methane and hydrogen. Poorly digested sulfur-rich proteins, found in beans, onions, garlic, eggs, and meat, produce the odor-iferous gases.

If soybeans are a regular food in your diet, it is important to make sure that they are thoroughly cooked before eating them. Uncooked soybeans contain a trypsin inhibitor that impedes the digestion of protein.

When a person ends a fast, or dramatically changes his or her diet, the pancreas must adapt to the new conditions by adjusting its secretion of digestive enzymes. For example, when a person eats a high-protein diet, the pancreas secretes up to seven times the normal amount of digestive enzymes capable of breaking down protein. Likewise, if the diet is exceptionally high in starch, the pancreas will secrete up to ten times the necessary amount of amylase. To minimize the stress of change, I recommend that a person alter their diet slowly, not overnight.

Stress

It is important to remember that the process of digestion begins even before we take our first bite of food. As we see and smell the food and think positive thoughts about it, digestive enzymes are already being secreted in the mouth and hydrochloric acid in the stomach. This is known as the cephalic phase of digestion, when the mind and senses trigger the body to prepare to receive food.

However, when a person is stressed, these responses are inhibited. Someone who is upset at mealtime may not be able to secrete enough acid or digestive enzymes, and this negative cephalic response can cause poor digestion.

A study published in *Digestive Diseases and Sciences* assessed the effect of acute mental stress on the secretion of pancreatic enzymes. Working with twelve healthy fasting volunteers, the researchers had each volunteer swallow tubing, which was then passed through the stomach and into the duodenum (upper intestine). The tubing allowed the researchers to monitor each volunteer's output of pancreatic chymotrypsin.

In order to induce mental stress, the volunteers were asked to perform mental arithmetic and solve anagrams for one hour. During the first half hour, there was no significant change in the average chymotrypsin concentration in the duodenum. However, during the second half hour, the concentration of chymotrypsin increased by 74 percent. In a thirty-minute period following the stressful activity, chymotrypsin concentration dropped precipitously, by 42 percent.

Managing stress can do much to improve digestive problems caused by low enzyme production. It is very important to take a moment before starting a meal to relax and prepare to enjoy the foods you are about to eat. When you are calm, you can better savor the flavors and textures of the foods being served as well as receive the health benefits that relaxed eating confers.

Pancreatic disease

The pancreas is very sensitive to the negative effects of certain drugs, alcohol, caffeine, and gallbladder disease. All of these factors can predispose an individual to pancreatitis, an inflammatory condition of the pancreas. Pancreatitis can manifest itself in two ways, depending on the speed and intensity of the disturbance. It can manifest in an acute form, known as acute pancreatitis, and in a slower, more insidious form, known as chronic pancreatitis. Both diseases impact pancreatic digestive-enzyme production.

Acute pancreatitis. The principal cause of acute pancreatitis in persons under fifty is alcoholism; but for older patients, the principal cause is cholelithiasis (gallstones). Younger patients tend to be men, whereas older patients are more likely to be women.

The acute form of pancreatitis is characterized by the sudden onset of severe episodes of abdominal pain. The pain is usually located in the region over the pit of the stomach (epigastrium) but may progress and involve the entire abdomen. It is almost invariably accompanied by nausea and vomiting, and fever is often also present.

Acute pancreatitis is characterized by inflammation. Normally, digestive enzymes in the pancreas are stored in a kind of protective shell, in an inactive form, and are only activated when needed in the intestinal tract. In acute pancreatitis, these digestive enzymes are suddenly activated and released within the pancreas itself. Trypsin (a protein-digesting enzyme) begins to break down the pancreas tissue, leading, over time, to the destruction of this organ.

Chronic pancreatitis. With some individuals, acute pancreatitis can progress to a chronic, recurring form. This is often seen in alcoholics. Individuals at high risk often have an intake of alcohol averaging thirteen ounces of liquor or two bottles or more of wine a day.

Symptoms, which can last days to weeks, include constant abdominal pain with nausea and vomiting. The interval between attacks may progressively shorten until the pain becomes almost continuous. There may be mild jaundice, with dark urine, fat in the stool, or symptoms of diabetes.

As the disease progresses, it causes irreversible damage to the pancreas with severe consequences to the health of individuals affected. Supplementation with pancreatic enzymes may be necessary in people with chronic pancreatic disease since their own production of enzymes is impaired with the destruction of the pancreatic tissue.

Many people largely ignore digestive distress for years, often treating their symptoms with over-the-counter remedies. By the time they are finally uncomfortable enough to seek medical care, a serious condition like pancreatic insufficiency or even pancreatic cancer may have developed.

When symptoms begin to occur and are not readily treatable with over-the-counter medication, or persist despite these medications, it is important to see your physician for a diagnostic evaluation. Be sure that your physician does a complete diagnostic workup including an assessment of pancreatic function.

If pancreatic and additional digestive functions are showing signs of impairment, it is crucial to begin a therapeutic program, implementing any needed dietary changes as well as the use of digestive enzymes and any nutritional supplements necessary to restore the health of your digestive tract.

The Aging Process

Pancreatic and other digestive-enzyme production is normally at its peak in children and young adults. But by the time most people reach their forties and fifties, the biochemical aging of the body begins to accelerate and the production of digestive enzymes diminishes.

Peak performance attributes such as the ability to absorb and assimilate food, the ability to suppress inflammation due to injury or disease, or even the ability to ward off the development of cancer begin to be compromised. I frequently hear from my patients that foods that were formerly easy to digest suddenly cause digestive distress.

Not only does digestive-enzyme production diminish with age, but all other digestive processes also become less efficient. There is reduced motility of the intestines, which hinders the ability to move food through the digestive tract, increasing transit time (the time it takes for a meal to be thoroughly digested and to pass from the body as feces) and making it more likely that a person will experience cramps, bloating, gas, constipation, diverticulosis (weakening of the intestinal wall), and perhaps even colon cancer.

With age, the stomach produces less hydrochloric acid, which assists protein digestion by activating pepsin, a digestive enzyme necessary for the breakdown of protein. Hydrochloric acid encourages the flow of bile and pancreatic digestive enzymes and facilitates the absorption of a variety of nutrients, including folic acid, vitamin C, beta-carotene, iron, calcium, magnesium, and zinc.

It also prevents bacterial and fungal overgrowth of the small intestine. Research studies have found that 30 percent of men and women in the United States over the age of 60 have atrophic gastritis, a condition in which little or no acid is secreted by the stomach, and that 40 percent of postmenopausal women have diminished gastric acid secretion.

There is, however, a great deal of variation as to the age at which symptoms of pancreatic—and, more generally, digestive—aging begin to manifest themselves. Symptoms of compromised digestive function can occur as early as the childhood or teen years or as late as the eighth or ninth decade of life—or even never, for digestive peak performers.

Whenever the symptoms of diminished pancreatic function appear, it is crucial that the problem be identified and pancreatic function restored for the continued health and well-being of the individual.

Even digestive peak performers can finally lose their ability to efficiently digest virtually anything they eat and convert their food into usable energy when they reach old age. Older people in their eighties, nineties, or even hundreds, who have always enjoyed robust health, excellent digestive function, and abundant energy, may find that even they must finally adopt an easier-to-digest diet.

When pancreatic-enzyme production diminishes to the point where individuals begin to experience symptoms that interfere with their ability to function adequately in important areas of their lives, they often seek medical help. These individuals often complain about a reduction in their energy level, decreased mental acuity, or painful inflammatory conditions. Many of them are concerned that their symptoms will interfere with their ability to earn a living and lead a full and varied life.

When I take a health history from such individuals, I find that they are often too tired to participate in many of their usual activities, such as their normal exercise routine or their usual round of social activities. They will spend more time at home and rest for longer periods of time. As their energy level diminishes, people begin to reduce their expectations of what they are capable of doing or achieving.

Luckily, one's diet can be modified to include more supplemental digestive enzymes and enzyme-rich foods available in pharmacies and health food stores can help to restore physical and mental energy by improving the absorption and assimilation of nutrients. These supplements are discussed in detail later on in this book.

Summary

The passage of time eventually affects the amount of pancreatic enzymes we produce, but diet and lifestyle are also important factors. The standard American diet, a high level of stress, and the overuse of alcohol, caffeine, and drugs all adversely affect the enzyme production of the pancreas.

4

Pancreatic Enzymes and Peak Performance

Abundant pancreatic digestive-enzyme production helps to maintain our physical and mental energy, as well as our productivity on the job. It also allows for varied and pleasurable social and business entertaining. Equally important, sufficient production of pancreatic enzymes is necessary for the prevention of and speedy recovery from minor illnesses, sprains, strains, and even injuries incurred in the workplace.

Physical Vitality and Stamina

Abundant physical and mental energy are important for success in any endeavor. The production of adequate pancreatic enzymes is a crucial link in the production of energy within the body. The link between healthy digestive function and physical and mental energy is not simply a modern concept, originating in Western medicine. It has been accepted for thousands of years in traditional healing models such as Asian medicine and the ancient Indian healing system of Ayurvedic medicine. In these models, individuals with weak digestive function are much more likely to be devitalized and fatigued.

Success in any career depends on having a high level of either physical or mental energy, or both. Abundant pancreatic-enzyme production is needed to assist the body in producing the energy needed to perform at an optimal level at one's job.

For example, most professional athletes eat enormous amounts of food in order to meet the energy demands of their nearly constant physical exertion. Abundant pancreatic-enzyme production is needed to convert the large amounts of calories that these individuals consume into usable energy, as well as to help maintain their body mass.

Only digestive peak performers can eat steaks, pizza, or several chicken breasts on a daily basis and turn this food into the energy they need to compete in major athletic events. In contrast, people with low pancreatic-enzyme production would normally feel tired and even suffer from indigestion after eating such foods, much less be able to go out and play a professional football, basketball, or baseball game.

Pancreatic enzymes are also among our body's most potent natural anti-inflammatory substances, they provide professional athletes with another benefit: the ability to recover quickly from traumatic injuries incurred during either competitive events or games or practice sessions. They also enable athletes to recover from periods of hard physical exertion and be able to compete effectively the following day.

Many nonathletic professions also require a high level of physical energy for success. For example, business people who travel frequently, entertainers on tour and politicians who are campaigning on the road all require vitality, stamina, and the ability to convert the food eaten on airplanes and in hotel restaurants into usable energy. Emergency room doctors, entrepreneurs doing start-ups and a myriad of other professions require enormous outputs of energy that healthy enzyme production helps to support.

Mental Clarity and Acuity

Mental acuity and sharpness depend as much as physical energy on adequate pancreatic-enzyme production. Our brains use 20 percent of our body's total energy. The millions of individuals who are engaged in careers requiring a high level of cognitive function depend, for their very livelihood, on a constant and abundant source of energy from the food that they ingest. Thus, peak performance in any intellectual endeavor is dependent on healthy digestive function as well as native intelligence.

Scientists, researchers, authors, and physicians, have very high energy requirements for their intellectually demanding work, which they are able to fulfill, in part, because of their healthy digestive function. I have found a surprising number of these individuals eat what would be considered medically unhealthy diets. Yet, like professional athletes, they are able to digest and convert the food they eat into the high level of mental energy that their demanding careers require without any obvious signs of pancreatic weakness, such as indigestion or inflammatory diseases.

The Ability to Get Along with Other People

Many of our social interactions involve the sharing of meals with our business associates, friends, and family. Sufficient digestive-enzyme production is necessary for successful participation in these gatherings.

Diminished pancreatic-enzyme production can limit the range and types of social interactions in which you can participate and even reduce the number of people with whom you feel comfortable spending time. A person with weak digestive function may instinctively avoid unfamiliar settings and cuisines, limiting their travels and experience to more comfortable settings, which they can count on not to stress their limited digestive capabilities.

For example, the capacity to enjoy many different types of cuisine is almost a prerequisite for a political career. You shouldn't even think of going into politics if you don't have a tremendous digestive capability and a cast-iron stomach.

Every politician on the campaign trail has to eat the food of the constituency that he or she is trying to attract. This can mean eating knishes in the Jewish neighborhood, egg rolls in the Chinese section of town, and kielbasa in the Polish neighborhood. I have seen photos of politicians stuffing down huge Subway sandwiches with ease while on the road campaigning.

Likewise, those individuals engaged in careers that require frequent socializing—such as public relations, sales, and even the diplomatic corps—face similar challenges as they attend endless rounds of cocktail parties, banquets, and other formal occasions where rich and hard-to-digest food is the staple.

Business people whose work requires them to travel frequently often face the same challenges. Business travel often includes lavish meals given or sponsored by the visitor or host. It is not unusual to have business meetings preceded or followed by a large breakfast buffet, lunch at the country club, and dinner at the new restaurant in town—three large, hard-to-digest meals in one day.

Executives working abroad must adapt not only to foreign foods, but also to different traditions surrounding meals. In Spain, little plates of hors d'oeuvres called tapas are served all evening, with dinner not served until eleven o'clock or midnight. In the Middle East, dinner is also eaten later in the evening.

Eating late can be very stressful for someone with marginally functional digestive capability. The digestive organs need to rest at night, and going to bed on a full stomach can leave a person feeling exhausted the next morning.

A patient of mine attended a Persian wedding at which only nuts and dried fruits were served during the hours before midnight. The actual wedding dinner, a lavish buffet with many highly spiced dishes, was served at 1:30 a.m. This heavy meal was a challenge to my patient; she needed to get up early in the morning and be fresh and alert for her job.

If your job or social life involves frequent attendance at events that include hard-to-digest food, be sure to load up on the enzyme-rich salads, fresh fruit, and vegetable side dishes. Avoid the heavy meat courses, butter, cheese, and desserts, which put excessive strain on the pancreas (leave those foods for the digestive peak performers).

In addition, the regular consumption of supplemental digestive enzymes both before and during your meal when attending banquets, cocktail parties, and other festive events can help you to prevent indigestion and maintain your energy level, allowing you to enjoy these events more. I'll discuss more about this important topic later on in this book.

Summary

Because of their role in helping to provide the body with energy, pancreatic enzymes are essential for anyone wanting to perform at the peak of their ability. Abundant enzyme production allows us to be at our best in the world of work and in social interactions.

5

Speedy Recovery from Illness, Injury, and Exertion

One of the hallmarks of peak performance is the ability to recover rapidly from physical stresses of all sorts, whether due to illness, physical exertion, long periods of immobility, accidents, injury, or even surgical procedures.

Abundant production of pancreatic enzymes helps the body to heal more rapidly from the inflammation caused by virtually any physical trauma, and reduces the stiffness and achiness that occur after exercise or even after long hours of sitting at a computer or in a car or airplane while traveling.

The important role that abundant pancreatic-enzyme production confers is dramatically illustrated by healthy children. Not only do children have the abundant digestive enzyme production that allows them to eat pizza, hamburgers, potato chips, ice cream, and cake, all at the same meal (a feat that few adults over the age of fifty can do without indigestion), but their strong pancreatic function also allows them to heal rapidly.

They are able to recover quickly from the falls, spills, and tumbles that occur while playing games and participating in sports. Children also remain active all day, moving from one activity to another, and experience very little, if any, stiffness or soreness the following day.

Similarly, adults who maintain a higher level of pancreatic digestive-enzyme production are more likely to be able to stay active and recover reasonably quickly from a weekend athletic event or from sitting in a cramped position on an airplane during a seventeen-hour international flight.

Unfortunately, most people lose their rapid-recovery capability as their pancreatic digestive-enzyme production begins to diminish at midlife. Very few adults enjoy this wonderful capacity.

In my practice, I hear a continuous list of complaints about aches, pains, and stiffness from my middle-aged and older patients. Even my twenty-year old friends complain about aches and pains when they do a lot of strenuous activities.

Luckily, the use of supplemental digestive enzymes can shorten recovery time and help limit the effects of injuries incurred from athletic activities or other types of physical trauma in the many individuals who have lost this important peak-performance function. The use of digestive enzymes can also help to reduce joint and muscle stiffness and achiness during periods of prolonged travel.

Sports Injuries

The benefits that supplemental pancreatic digestive enzymes provide in helping to limit the extent of traumatic injury and in promoting healing are so well known in sports medicine that they are routinely used in America and abroad by athletes at all levels of competition, both prophylactically and as part of treatment once a bruise or rupture of tissue has occurred.

Numerous studies confirm the effectiveness of pancreatic enzymes in treating sports injuries, regardless of the type of injury or its severity. In a study published in the *South African Medical Journal*, twenty-three patients with soft-tissue damage from sports injuries were given proteolytic-enzyme treatment.

Researchers noted patients on enzymes, compared to those not treated, experienced quicker recovery from bruising. Function of the injured site was restored more rapidly, and the athletes more quickly regained their fitness to resume play. The researchers suggested that the use of enzyme treatment to accelerate healing could be valuable in maintaining morale and personal fitness as well as performance skills.

In another study, appearing in *The British Journal of Clinical Practice*, 100 patients with fractures of the hand were divided into two groups, with one group receiving pancreatic-enzyme treatment and the other remaining untreated. The dosage was two tablets every four hours, taken half an hour before meals, for five days.

Researchers measured the subjects' ability to move the affected fingers, since this reflected the degree of swelling, pain, and function of the joint and tendon. Over 80 percent of those patients receiving enzymes showed a significant improvement in mobility, as compared with only 50 percent in the untreated group.

Further, in a pair of studies conducted at a clinic in Wiesbaden, Germany, and presented at the FIMS World Congress of Sports Medicine, pancreatic enzymes were given to patients undergoing surgery for sports injuries.

In the first study, 80 patients having knee surgery were divided into two groups, one treated with enzymes postoperatively. These patients experienced a significantly more rapid reduction in edema (retention of fluid in the tissues) and a more rapid return to complete mobility.

In the second study, 120 patients who were undergoing surgical treatment of fractures were divided into two groups. The patients in one group received enzyme treatment, beginning five days before the operation. Treated patients had significantly less preoperative edema and notably less pain and edema on the day of the operation.

In a comparison of the two studies, the researcher concluded that enzyme treatment was most beneficial when begun before admission to the hospital, as it reduces symptoms, better prepares the patient for surgery, and allows patients to leave the hospital earlier.

Many professional athletes use pancreatic enzymes prophylactically, anticipating that they will sustain physical wear and tear during a sporting event. They cannot afford to sustain an injury that would debilitate them or force them to curtail their playing time. Periods of forced inactivity can mean large financial losses to highly paid athletes, their teams, and their sponsors if they miss tournaments, play-off games, or infrequent events like the Olympics.

In a clinical trial published in *The Practitioner*, 494 boxers with cuts, hematomas (blood clots), bruising, superficial laceration, and sprains of the finger joints were given enzyme treatment. Half of the group took enzymes before boxing, while the rest were given a placebo.

Prophylactic use of the enzyme preparation resulted in a fifty percent reduction in bruising and an eleven percent reduction in the incidence of hematomas. Boxers who received lacerations were able to return to the ring as soon as one to two weeks after injury, as opposed to the four weeks that it normally takes to recover from such trauma. Hematomas and bruises treated with enzymes resolved even more rapidly, clearing in just four to five days.

The results of these studies suggest that taking enzymes prophylactically (before the event, as a preventive measure) or while engaging in an intense physical activity offers great benefit for those people who engage in sporadic intense physical exertion.

I recommend that several days before engaging in competitive athletic activities that require maximum effort (like a fun run) or physical contact (like touch football or pickup basketball games) or that result in unavoidable falls (like skiing, skateboarding, or rollerblading), take supplemental digestive enzymes.

The same advice holds for those who enjoy active vacations centered on skiing, bicycling, or hiking. Likewise, for those who engage in intense activities such as gardening, shoveling snow, or strenuous home repair. Following a program of using enzymes prophylactically or therapeutically can reduce or eliminate day-after stiffness or soreness.

Baby boomers are particularly prone to accidents and injuries while engaging in strenuous physical activity. In fact, sports-related injuries in individuals between the ages of forty and sixty-four have increased by more than 20 percent over the past few decades.

This is due in part to the tendency of baby boomers to resist the notion of their own physical aging. They often balance their intense work schedules with sporadic, aggressive physical exercise.

If you do sustain an accident or injury, immediately begin an aggressive program of enzyme supplementation using a combination of bromelain, papain, and/or pancreatic enzymes (see chapter 9 for specific recommendations) to reduce the inflammation and facilitate the repair process. Continue this program until the inflammation is eliminated and the injury is healed. You will be back in action much sooner and have less downtime, especially as you get older.

Repetitive Stress Injuries

According to a statement by the administrator of the Occupational Safety and Health Administration that appeared in an issue of the *OSHA Compliance News*, the fastest-growing occupational health hazard in the United States is injury resulting from repetitive stress. The growth rate of these injuries is so rapid that the National Institute for Occupational Safety and Health predicted that approximately fifty percent of the workforce would suffer some form of cumulative trauma disorder (CTD) by the year 2000.

CTD is an umbrella term that includes all types of work-related repetitive-stress injuries to the muscles, nerves, and tendons of the upper body. The medical conditions that develop from repetitive stress are chronic back pain, frozen shoulder, tendonitis, bursitis, epicondylitis (also known as tennis or golfer's elbow), and carpal tunnel syndrome, the wrist disorder that can cause numbness, tingling, and severe, incapacitating pain.

In addition, chronic conditions that typically impair performance on the job, such as osteoarthritis and rheumatoid arthritis, are also worsened by repetitive stress.

Repetitive-stress injuries are incurred in occupations or fields as diverse as computer programming or data entry, meat cutting and packing, assembly line work, grocery scanning, painting, telemarketing, and dental hygiene.

The parts of the body affected by these conditions tend to become chronically inflamed, with pain and swelling at the primary location of the injury. Many hobbies, such as knitting and sewing, and sports activities, such as tennis and golf, require repetitive motions, so their practitioners may also be prone to these types of injuries.

The economic costs of these CTDs are very high. *BusinessWeek* magazine reports that the lost earnings and medical costs of these injuries are in excess of $27 billion annually. For carpal tunnel syndrome alone, the costs of medical treatment, surgical procedures, lost time from work, and rehabilitation expenses are estimated to be $25,000 to $60,000 per incidence.

For many people, the injuries are so debilitating that they are unable to continue with their current jobs or to participate in their favorite sports for prolonged periods of time.

Unfortunately, very little emphasis has been placed on healing the damage caused by repetitive-stress injuries. Most people who alter or eliminate the repetitive motions that caused the injury are still unable to reduce or eliminate the pain, swelling, and discomfort in the affected area.

In all of these cases, digestive enzymes can play a powerful healing role. Pancreatic enzymes and plant-based enzymes such as bromelain and papain, which are discussed later on in this book, are very effective anti-inflammatory agents. Used aggressively, these enzymes can be very effective in reducing pain at the site of the injury and promoting healing and recovery of function.

The therapeutic benefit of enzymes was corroborated in an interesting medical study published in *Clinical Medicine* of individuals suffering from tenosynovitis of their arms due to injury incurred in their work, which required repetitive motion for many hours each day. Symptoms resolved much more rapidly in workers who were treated with digestive enzymes than in untreated workers.

Individuals with repetitive-stress injuries or joint or muscle conditions aggravated by repetitive stress will heal more readily if supplemental digestive enzymes are taken as often as 4 times per day until symptoms begin to resolve.

Minor Surgery and Dental Procedures

Another area where enzymes can play a significant role in healing and recovery time is before and after minor outpatient surgeries and dental procedures, which have increased dramatically in recent years.

According to the U.S. National Center for Health Statistics, there are many millions of outpatient operations performed in hospitals and freestanding surgical centers (not including dentistry, abortions, podiatry, birthing, family planning, pain blocks, or other small procedures). Similarly, patients undergo millions of dental surgeries and tooth extractions each year.

While considered minor, these operations and procedures can cause a great deal of pain, swelling, and discomfort, with recovery times lasting up to seven days. However, by using enzymes both pre- and postoperatively, the inflammatory response is significantly diminished, lessening pain and swelling and enhancing the body's ability to heal.

Acute illnesses, trauma from surgical procedures or repetitive-stress injuries incurred while participating in sports or on the job, should be treated aggressively with digestive enzymes to limit inflammation and promote rapid and efficient healing.

Begin enzyme therapy several days prior to surgery or immediately once an acute illness or repetitive-stress injury begins to become symptomatic. These conditions should never be allowed to proceed to a chronic state, where recovery is much more prolonged and difficult to achieve.

Enzymes can be used in conjunction with any prescribed antibiotics, painkillers, or hot or cold compresses. The immediate therapeutic use of digestive enzymes can save people weeks or even months of disability and pain.

Summary

Because of their role in helping to reduce trauma and injury, pancreatic enzymes are essential for anyone wanting to speeds recovery from physical trauma. This can include work and sports related injury and surgery.

6

Digestive Enzyme Production and Health

While pancreatic digestive enzymes are very useful in maintaining many aspects of peak performance, they can also play an important role in the treatment of various health problems. The benefits of abundant digestive-enzyme production in assisting rapid recovery from accidents, injury and surgery were discussed in the previous chapter. They are also useful in combating a variety of other inflammatory conditions, as I will discuss in this chapter.

Colds, Flus, Bronchitis, Sinusitis, and Allergies

Peak performance—and even the ability to just show up at work or social engagements—is significantly hampered by common respiratory illnesses. Millions of Americans, both children and adults, suffer from as many as four to six colds per year, or have allergy symptoms to common triggers such as pollens, grasses, and mold that can drag on for months. The symptoms that accompany these conditions can seriously hamper a person's ability to fulfill their job or household and family responsibilities; much less perform at optimal levels.

Although considered minor illnesses, colds, flus, bronchitis, and allergies often force those affected to take time off from work or abstain from athletics or social activities. Moreover, colds and flus are one of the most common reasons for children to miss school, and constant absenteeism due to these conditions can greatly hamper a child's ability to learn and keep up with the rest of the class.

In my practice, I often see people who have had acute sinus conditions, colds, and flus that have taken anywhere from two to six weeks to be completely resolved, despite the use of prescription or over-the-counter drugs, which often simply substitute one set of lingering symptoms for another and do not cure the underlying causes. These conditions are truly major success saboteurs.

There are four functions necessary for combating colds, flus, bronchitis, sinusitis, middle-ear infections, and allergies: good buffering capability (the ability to alkalinize), the ability to suppress inflammation with the production of pancreatic enzymes, healthy detoxification, and the ability to keep our cells and tissues well oxygenated. In this chapter, I'll discuss the role of enzymes in limiting infection.

The highly acidic, inflammatory diet most Americans eat plays a major role in triggering respiratory infections and allergies. When respiratory tissues are inflamed from either infection or allergy, the result is nasal congestion, sore throat, swollen and painful sinuses, itching and tearing of the eyes, fluid in the middle ears, and excess bronchial secretions that lead to coughing.

Unfortunately, while over-the-counter drugs can help to suppress coughs, reduce fever, and dry up nasal congestion, they often produce equally unpleasant side effects such as racing heart, drowsiness, and feeling light-headed or drugged.

One of the most effective methods to suppress respiratory inflammation is by taking supplemental pancreatic enzymes as well as other natural anti-inflammatory substances such as plant-based digestive enzymes like papain, which is derived from papayas, and bromelain, which is derived from pineapples.

One study, published in *Drugs Under Experimental and Clinical Research*, examined the therapeutic effect of a plant-based digestive enzyme product used in combination with an antibiotic on patients with respiratory illnesses such as chronic bronchitis and pneumonia.

The addition of the digestive enzyme to the treatment regimen improved the absorption of the antibiotics and increased their level in the lungs, thereby improving the efficacy of the antibiotics. In addition, more of the patients on enzyme therapy had total resolution of their symptoms. There were also far fewer patients who failed to respond to the combined therapy than to drug treatment alone.

Enzyme therapy was found to reduce inflammation of the respiratory tissue and to help suppress coughing. In a clinical study involving patients with chronic bronchitis, reduction of coughing was noted after ten days of enzyme therapy.

Another research study found that 87 percent of patients undergoing treatment for sinusitis with digestive-enzyme therapy had a significant reduction of their symptoms. I have seen similar results in my own practice, with many patients experiencing dramatic relief from long-standing sinus conditions after using supplemental digestive enzymes.

A Guide to Rapid Recovery from Colds and Flus

I know two digestive peak performers who have described their amazingly quick recovery from colds, runny noses, and sore throats during the past year. I want to share their program with you because it is so effective.

At the first signs of a cold or flu, they leave the office and go home to take a rest or nap and eat lightly and go to bed early. They are normally able to resolve their symptoms rapidly and without the use of drugs and be back at the top of their game in one to two days rather than the two to six weeks that many other people require.

Their instinctive, and obviously successful, strategy in dealing with these minor illnesses plays to their innate strength. They allow the digestive enzymes that they both abundantly produce to reduce the signs of respiratory inflammation. By immediately reducing their food intake, they can use their digestive enzymes to reduce inflammation instead of to digest a rich meal.

These individuals also tend to be naturally alkaline; therefore, they have excellent buffering capability and are able to neutralize the excess acidity seen with infection and allergies, and their strong immune systems are able to overcome any exposure to bacteria or viruses.

If you tend to produce low levels of pancreatic enzymes and are prone to colds, flus, sinusitis, middle-ear infections, bronchitis, and allergies, it is very helpful to use supplemental digestive enzymes at the first sign of any of these conditions.

To get the most benefit from these powerful anti-inflammatory enzymes, eat lightly for the first twelve to forty-eight hours after the onset of symptoms, mostly soups and steamed vegetables. In addition, be sure to reduce your level of activity and rest or nap. Finally, consume large amounts of water.

These measures should help to significantly reduce your symptoms in one to two days. In addition, improving your acid/alkaline balance, promoting healthy detoxification, and following a program to increase the oxygen levels within your cells and tissues will help to improve your resistance to respiratory conditions.

If you are prone to respiratory conditions and tend to travel frequently, or are involved in stressful work or recreational activities, be sure to always have an emergency kit with you that contains supplemental digestive enzymes as well as the other cold remedies described in this book, such as colloidal silver, sodium and potassium bicarbonate, and anti-infectious and anti-inflammatory herbs such as echinacea and ginger.

Food Allergies

The allergic reactions that millions of people experience in response to certain foods as well as environmental allergens such as mold, dust, trees, and pollen can cause uncomfortable and even debilitating symptoms.

Common foods such as milk, wheat, eggs, and peanuts can seriously impair the performance capability of affected individuals. Intestinal cramps, food intolerances, brain fog, fatigue, poor physical stamina and endurance, emotional and behavioral upsets, and a variety of other physical symptoms can occur in response to eating foods that one is allergic to.

Digestive enzymes can help to reduce the allergic reactions that some people have to certain foods. When a person lacks sufficient digestive enzymes, large molecules of incompletely digested protein can be absorbed through the small intestine and trigger an allergic reaction.

The immune system is unable to respond appropriately and reacts to improperly digested food as a foreign substance, which can initiate an allergic, inflammatory reaction. This occurs either directly at the intestinal wall or creates a systemic reaction, resulting in fatigue, inflammation and swelling in various tissues like the joints or thyroid, headaches, or even psychiatric disturbances.

As we age, there is a greater likelihood of developing allergic reactions to various foods as the production of anti-inflammatory digestive enzymes diminishes. I often see patients in their forties and fifties who had previously been able to eat wheat or dairy products (statistically, two of the most allergy-producing foods) suddenly become unable to tolerate them.

While this is a reasonably common occurrence as people reach midlife, it can also occur in much younger individuals. Many young children, teenagers, and adults in their twenties and thirties have food allergies. Research studies have linked food allergies to conditions that typically affect younger individuals such as attention deficit disorder, chronic fatigue, behavioral disorders, and respiratory conditions.

All of these conditions can impair the performance capability of younger individuals, affecting their ability to learn, enjoy good social relations, and even participate in the type of vigorous physical activity that healthy children and young adults normally participate in.

Allergies can also be an underlying cause of chronic-fatigue symptoms. Psychiatrists who have done research in the area of nutrition and mental health have even suggested that food allergies may trigger schizophrenia and other mental aberrations. The use of supplemental digestive enzymes is a very important part of any treatment program for individuals with food allergies.

Inflammatory Diseases

Inflammation and its accompanying pain are a major component of a number of diseases, including food allergies, rheumatoid arthritis, interstitial cystitis, Crohn's disease, endometriosis, and colitis. Because pancreatic digestive enzymes help to reduce inflammation, they can be a useful part of the treatment program. While all inflammatory diseases are characterized clinically by pain, heat, swelling, and discomfort, the specific symptoms vary depending on the type of tissue affected.

Rheumatoid arthritis

Research on the benefits of enzymes for the treatment of rheumatoid arthritis has been done in Europe, particularly Germany, where enzymes have been found to be effective in reducing such common symptoms as stiffness, swelling, pain, and limited mobility.

Rheumatic disease is characterized by increases in the presence of immune complexes. Circulating immune complexes (CICs) form when viruses, bacteria, toxic chemicals, and overly large molecules of protein are absorbed into the systemic circulation. These foreign substances stimulate the immune system to produce antibodies, which act as the body's SWAT team. They are shaped like the letter Y and bind to substances they come into contact with. The resulting compounds are known as circulating immune complexes large aggregates or clumps of foreign cells (antigens) and antibodies.

While CICs can be free-floating in the blood, sometimes they are deposited in tissue. Once in tissues, they can trigger an inflammatory response, leading to localized tissue destruction. Elevated levels of CICs have been reported in patients suffering from rheumatoid arthritis, Crohn's disease, lupus, and thyroiditis.

A study published in *Biomedicine & Pharmacotherapy* found that digestive-enzyme treatment can be used successfully to destroy these complexes, thereby neutralizing their detrimental effect on the various tissues of the body, including the joints.

I have worked with many arthritis patients, ranging from a preteen boy to a woman in her eighties. However, this condition is more common in women, particularly after midlife. Most of these patients have responded well to nutritional therapy.

One such case was a fifty-three-year-old female technical writer who was diagnosed with rheumatoid arthritis two years after going through a difficult menopause. Her job, which required extensive use of a computer, had become extremely difficult due to the pain and swelling in the joints of her hands. She was concerned that her symptoms would make it impossible for her to continue a career that she was both proficient at and enjoyed.

However, after several months of nutritional therapy, including dietary modification and the use of digestive enzymes, along with conventional therapy (which had been only moderately helpful on its own), she found that the swelling and pain in her hands greatly subsided.

Crohn's disease

Crohn's disease is another health condition for which the therapeutic use of pancreatic enzymes can produce significant benefits. Similar to those with rheumatoid arthritis, patients with Crohn's disease test positive for the presence of circulating immune complexes. The extent of the damage these CICs cause within tissue can be limited by the use of digestive enzymes.

In Crohn's disease, the affected tissue is usually within the small intestine, primarily the terminal part called the ileum. These tissues can become chronically inflamed and irritated. As the inflamed tissues heal, they can form scar tissue that narrows the intestinal passageway. The onset of the disease is typically around the age of twenty; symptoms include diarrhea, periodic cramping, lower right abdominal pain, fever, malabsorption, possible anemia, a lack of energy, poor appetite, and weight loss.

Endometriosis

A relatively common problem, endometriosis affects 7 to 15 percent of the female population of the United States. Cells comprising the lining of the uterus, called the endometrium, break away and grow outside the uterine cavity, implanting themselves in many locations within the pelvis, including the ovaries, ligaments of the uterus, cervix, appendix, bowel, and bladder.

Endometriosis causes inflammation and scarring in the pelvis, resulting in chronic pain and discomfort. Elevated estrogen levels in the body stimulate the growth of these implants with each menstrual cycle. Thus, lowering the level of estrogen within the body is needed to limit the growth and spread of this condition.

In addition, controlling the inflammation within the pelvis is equally important if a woman suffering from this condition is to achieve symptom relief. The use of natural anti-inflammatory agents like digestive enzymes can be quite helpful in this regard.

A study noted in the *American Journal of Obstetrics and Gynecology* found that two plant-based digestive enzymes, papain and bromelain, were quite useful for the relief of menstrual pain.

An additional study, published in *Drugs Under Experimental and Clinical Research*, examined the tissue penetration of several antibiotic drugs and indomethacin, an anti-inflammatory medication, in women with a variety of gynecological complaints, including fibroid tumors of the uterus and ovarian cysts. Some of the women were also given bromelain as part of a controlled study.

After administration of the drugs with or without bromelain, all of the women underwent surgical removal of reproductive tissue to treat their primary conditions. The study found that when bromelain was administered concurrently with antibiotics, the absorption and tissue penetration of the antibiotics were significantly increased.

This was found to be true in all of the reproductive tissue examined after surgery, including the uterus, fallopian tubes, and ovaries. Enzyme therapy can also benefit male reproductive function. Anti-inflammatory digestive enzymes can also be used to reduce the swelling and pain that occur with prostatitis.

Vascular Disease

Heart attacks and strokes are caused by obstruction in the arterial blood vessels due to atherosclerosis, which blocks the normal flow of blood to the heart and brain. Atherosclerosis is described as a condition by deposits of cholesterol on the inner layer of the arterial walls, which results in the formation of fibrous, fatty plaques.

Although most people are unaware that inflammation plays an important role in the development of these plaques, medical research has found a strong association between the development of heart disease and inflammation. The use of pancreatic enzymes can help to limit the inflammatory damage occurring within the blood vessels and to reduce the tendency of platelets to clump or aggregate. Platelets are a component of the blood necessary for normal clotting. The risk of heart attacks and strokes is increased when platelets become abnormally sticky and impair normal blood flow through the blood vessels.

Another risk factor for strokes and heart attacks is elevated levels of cholesterol and triglycerides. Research studies have found that treatment with digestive enzymes can reduce levels of these blood lipids.

A study published in *Atherosclerosis* examined eighty-four female volunteers, aged sixty-three to ninety-five, in a geriatric ward in a hospital in Sheffield, England. During a twenty-five day trial, half of the women received a daily enzyme preparation that included lipase, while the other volunteers were given a placebo.

On the day after admission to the trial, the volunteers were fed a high-fat, high-cholesterol meal that included eggs and cream. The researchers recorded the rise in the women's triglyceride and cholesterol levels following the fat-rich meal. This same procedure was repeated at the end of the trial, and changes in triglyceride levels and cholesterol were compared.

Levels of triglycerides after meals at the end of the study, as compared with levels at the start, were only 1.25 percent lower in the untreated women, while levels dropped 14.4 percent in those volunteers receiving enzymes. At the end of the trial, researchers also observed lower levels of cholesterol in those women receiving enzymes if their initial levels were relatively high. Elevated levels of cholesterol and triglycerides are big issues for a number of my patients and enzymes are a very exciting treatment option.

Enzyme therapy can also be useful in the treatment of venous thrombosis, a condition in which blood clots form most commonly within the veins of the legs, which can lead to a blockage or occlusion of the affected blood vessel. The greatest danger associated with these types of clots is that they can become detached and move through the circulatory system toward the heart or lungs and cause a life-threatening embolism.

Enzymes have also been found to be effective in treating post-thrombotic (clot related) leg ulcers. According to a study published in the *British Journal of Clinical Practice*, ten patients out of a group of nineteen, aged 32 to 87 were treated with an ointment containing protein-digesting enzymes. The other patients in the group were treated with an ointment containing an antibiotic-steroid formulation without enzymes.

After six weeks of treatment, ulcers receiving the enzyme treatment were more reduced in size and in two cases were completely healed. No comparable improvement was observed in the other group. Enzyme treatment has the further advantage of being relatively painless and requiring less nursing time.

Cancer

Cancer is such a terrifying and, even, life threatening disease for so many people, that it is great to know that digestive enzymes can have significant benefit in the treatment of this disease, too.

The anti-tumor effect of pancreatic enzymes was discovered at the turn of the century by John Beard, a highly respected embryologist at the University of Edinburgh Medical School. He reasoned that the placenta is, from one perspective, much like a cancer: It is foreign tissue that grows at a fast rate and is highly invasive. Theoretically, it should be rejected by the mother since half the genes in these cells are from the father, making the placenta genetically incompatible.

Then Beard made a remarkable discovery. He observed that in all mammals, the growth of the placenta stops on a certain day. This occurs in humans fifty-six days after conception. For decades, he searched for an explanation. What he found was that in both animals and humans, placental growth ceased when the fetal pancreas began to produce digestive enzymes. Beard concluded that these enzymes were the trigger that stopped the growth.

Based on this conclusion, he then set up experiments to test if the pancreatic enzymes also had a more generalized role of limiting or stopping uncontrolled growth in other parts of the body. Beard injected pancreatic extracts containing high levels of digestive enzymes directly into malignant tumors, treating a total of 170 cancer patients in this manner.

Using the enzyme-rich pancreatic digestive juices of newborn lambs, pigs, and calves, Beard found that more than half the patients with advanced cancer survived longer than expected, and in some patients, cancers disappeared completely.

Between 1902 and 1905, the use of enzymes in the treatment of cancer generated interest within the medical profession. But in 1905, Marie Curie was showing great progress in successfully shrinking tumors with radiation, and her work drew attention away from Beard's efforts. Enzyme therapy was eclipsed by this new work, and it wasn't until the 1960s that there was renewed interest in its benefits.

A current explanation of why pancreatic enzymes are able to reduce tumors is based on a particular defense mechanism of cancer cells. Cancer cells that escape initial attack and destruction by the immune system travel through the circulation and adhere to cell walls and multiply at various sites.

In order to avoid detection, they coat themselves with an adhesive fibrin layer fifteen times thicker than that of normal cells. Pancreatic enzymes are able to break down this fibrin layer, reducing inflammation and exposing the cancer cells. This allows the cancer cells to be more easily detected and destroyed by the immune system.

Today, a small number of modern physicians in the United States and Europe follow Beard's theories, prescribing pancreatic enzymes for the treatment of cancer. Like Beard, some of these physicians claim to be able to produce unusually long survival times in their pancreatic cancer patients.

In contrast, the cure rates for patients with pancreatic cancer undergoing conventional chemotherapy are abysmal. Most of these patients follow a very rapid downhill course, often dying within sixty to ninety days of diagnosis. (The use of enzymes in cancer treatment is discussed more fully later on in this book).

Summary

The production of abundant pancreatic enzymes not only helps to accelerate recovery from trauma, respiratory illnesses, and exertion, but can be useful in the treatment of a number of inflammatory diseases, vascular diseases, and possibly even cancer.

7

Evaluating your Own Levels of Digestive Enzymes

By now, you may be wondering about your own production of digestive enzymes, particularly if you have any of the conditions that I have previously discussed in this book. While the diagnosis of pancreatic insufficiency or disease requires medical testing, I have developed the following checklist so that you can do your own self-assessment on whether you may be suffering from a lack of digestive enzyme production.

The occurrence of the following symptoms on a chronic basis suggests that your enzyme production may be deficient. You can use the checklist as a tool to help you assess whether you need to begin to make some dietary changes and take digestive enzyme supplements as recommended in this book.

This checklist can also help you decide whether you should be evaluated by your doctor to determine if you have undetected disease. Your responses to this checklist can provide your physician with a useful tool for diagnosis and a starting point for your medical care.

There is no quantitative grading for this checklist, any of the symptoms listed could be an indicator of pancreatic disease or other digestive problems. If a number of these items apply, you should consult a health care professional and begin to implement a program to restore your digestive health.

Digestive Enzyme Self-Assessment Quiz

Performance indicators

Put a check mark beside those statements that are true for you.

- o I feel I am restricted in my ability to eat a wide variety of foods, either in business or social settings.
- o I experience a low level of energy despite eating adequate amounts of food.
- o I am slow to recover from injury.
- o I experience excessive stiffness and/or soreness the day after heavy exercise.
- o I tire easily from work or play.
- o I am unable to travel without great fatigue.
- o I have difficulty thinking clearly and quickly.

Lifestyle/environmental factors

- o I have a history of excessive alcohol intake.
- o I feel poorly on a diet high in fats, animal protein, and sugars.

Physical indicators

- o I often suffer from indigestion.
- o I frequently have abdominal bloating and discomfort after meals, a condition unrelieved by antacids.
- o I often experience intestinal cramps after eating.
- o I often experience flatulence after meals.
- o My food appears relatively undigested and greasy in the stools.
- o I suffer from chronic diarrhea.
- o I am frequently constipated, particularly after eating certain foods.
- o I have difficulty digesting highly spiced and unfamiliar foreign foods.
- o I often feel tired after a meal.

Medical history

- o I have a history of chronic pancreatitis.
- o I have a history of Crohn's disease, ulcerative colitis, or irritable-bowel syndrome.
- o I have had gallstones.
- o I suffer from rheumatoid arthritis.
- o I have a history of vasculitis.
- o I have a history of endometriosis.
- o I have food and environmental allergies.

Laboratory Tests to Assess Pancreatic and General Digestive Function

If you decide that you need to go further and work with your physician or health care provider for an in-depth laboratory evaluation of your digestive enzyme function, there are a number of tests available.

There are stool tests that allow physicians to accurately evaluate pancreatic digestive-enzyme production by measuring levels of enzymes in the stool, as well as monitoring such crucial digestive functions as the digestion of animal proteins, vegetable matter, and starch.

These tests also measure the presence of any excess fat in the stool (which is seen with weak pancreatic function), the maintenance of intestinal pH levels, and the adequacy of intestinal immune function.

Culturing is also done to monitor the presence of mucus, blood, and both normal and abnormal bacteria, yeast, and fungi.

Other tests measure the presence of enzymes in the urine and blood that can be elevated when there is inflammation of the pancreas. Pancreatitis and related gallbladder disease may also be assessed using ultrasound and X-rays.

Urinary analysis is helpful in assessing the health of the pancreas. With acute pancreatitis, there is increased urinary amylase, the result of spillage when the gland is damaged. Values exceeding five times the upper limit of normal are characteristic of acute pancreatitis. Because of intermittent elevations of amylase from hour to hour, a single specimen is inadequate; a two- or six-hour collection is more accurate.

Ultrasound testing, a method of imaging our internal organs, is a simple and noninvasive test to detect pancreatic disease. When pancreatitis is acute, an enlarged, inflamed pancreas is seen in 90 percent of cases. The pancreas will have an irregular shape, sometimes with a dilated pancreatic duct. In the case of acute pancreatitis caused by gallbladder disease, the physician may order an ultrasound of the upper abdomen, which is useful in visualizing the stones.

Part II:
Restoring Your Digestive Enzymes

In the following chapters, I will provide you with a very effective and easy-to-follow four-part plan to both improve your digestive capability and help restore your own production of digestive enzymes.

In Chapter 8, you will learn which foods supply enzymes in their natural state and how to best prepare these foods for optimal absorption and assimilation.

In Chapter 9, I provide you with much valuable information on pancreatic and digestive enzymes. The use of supplemental digestive enzymes will give you the immediate digestive firepower that you may have lost years ago or perhaps never had. You will also learn how to use these enzymes as powerful anti-inflammatory agents.

Chapter 10 will provide you with information about other natural anti-inflammatory substances that can be used in combination with digestive enzymes to treat a variety of inflammatory conditions.

Finally, chapter 11 provides information about other digestive aids that can be used to support proper absorption and assimilation of foods and nutrients in individuals with weak digestive function.

8

The Enzyme-Rich Diet

Foods that are rich in their own natural enzymes provide you with natural digestants and anti-inflammatory chemicals. In this way, the foods themselves aid in the process of digestion and ease the work of the pancreas. There are four steps to eating an enzyme-rich diet:

1. Choose enzyme-rich foods.
2. Avoid foods that stress the pancreas.
3. Drink blenderized beverages, if indicated.
4. Eat pureed foods if indicated.

I will now discuss each of these steps in detail.

Step 1: Choose Enzyme-Rich Foods

The best foods for an enzyme-rich diet are fresh fruits (particularly ones with low acid content like melons and papayas, if you tend to be overly acidic) and vegetables, along with sprouted beans and seeds. These foods are easy to digest because they contain natural enzymes and, if well chewed, do not create stress on the pancreas; they should be included with many of your meals.

Various plant enzymes assist in the ripening and maturation process as well as the eventual breakdown and decay of the plant. When raw plant foods are consumed, their enzymes assist in the breakdown of food, beginning in the upper digestive tract. As the food passes through the digestive tract, these plant enzymes ease the workload of the digestive system and reduce the demand on the body's store of enzymes. Over time, this assistance can have a restorative effect on the body's digestive capability.

Fresh Fruits and Vegetables

All fresh fruits and vegetables contain natural digestive enzymes. Two fruits in particular, pineapple and papaya, contain some of the most potent protein-digesting enzymes. The proteolytic enzyme in pineapple is bromelain, and in papaya, papain.

Of these two, papain is most useful as a digestive enzyme because of its soothing effect on the stomach. Bromelain is used as a potent anti-inflammatory. I may recommend to patients that they include papaya in their diet. However, many individuals with low enzyme production are also highly acidic, and pineapple and its juice are highly acidic and may cause canker sores and digestive upset in overly acidic individuals.

Therefore, I don't recommend eating pineapple except on an infrequent basis. Luckily, the best delivery system for these enzymes is in supplemental form, which allows one to benefit from the enzymatic properties of both fruits. Supplementation with papain and bromelain is addressed in detail in Chapter 9.

Sprouted Seeds, Grains, and Legumes

All sprouted seeds are exceptionally rich sources of natural enzymes. A seed that is in the process of sprouting is in a very active state of maturation, rich in enzymes and nutrients. When a seed sprouts, its nutrient value multiplies many times. Alfalfa sprouts contain as much beta-carotene as carrots, as well as high levels of calcium, iron, magnesium, potassium, phosphorus, sodium, sulfur, silicon, chlorine, cobalt, and zinc. Green peas, lentils, garbanzo beans, sunflower seeds, adzuki beans, and mung beans can all be sprouted. A wide variety of sprouts are available in local supermarkets as well as natural food stores and farmers' markets.

While all raw foods including fish, meat, and poultry contain enzymes, eating raw flesh foods can be very hazardous due to bacteria and parasites. This is especially true when you do not personally know how the meat, fish, or poultry has been handled since it was slaughtered or caught. Therefore, the eating of raw flesh foods, even though they retain their natural enzymes, is not encouraged.

It is important to know that cooked foods do not contain active enzymes. When food is heated above 140°F, all its valuable enzymes are destroyed. All common cooking techniques such as sautéing, frying, boiling, and baking occur at temperatures that are well in excess of this threshold. Even such reputedly healthy cooking techniques as steaming and slow cooking are commonly done at temperatures well above 140°F. All food that is canned or otherwise heat-processed has also lost all of its living enzymes and must rely on the enzymes created by the body for its digestion.

The cooking process also destroys certain amounts of vitamins, minerals, and other phytonutrients. Such foods may still have many healthy vitamins and minerals, all of its natural enzymes have been inactivated.

Frozen foods, usually considered healthier than canned foods, also retain virtually none of their active enzymes. Almost all frozen foods have been blanched (placed in boiling water for two to six minutes, depending on the fruit or vegetable) prior to freezing with the express purpose of arresting the enzyme activity so as to not bring about other nutritional losses or create off flavors through the activity of the natural enzymes.

Commercial fruit juices have been pasteurized, which also inactivates their enzymes. However, fresh juices made at home using a juicer retain the active enzymes found in the raw fruits and vegetables they are made from.

To significantly increase the level of nutrients and natural enzymes in your diet, add sprouted seeds and beans to your meals, for example, in salads or sandwiches. You may enjoy the taste of some sprouts more than others—so experiment. Try sprouted sunflower seeds, flaxseeds, radish, broccoli, onions, adzuki beans, garbanzo beans, and lentils. You can find sprouts in natural food stores and at farmers' markets.

All raw seeds, beans, and grains are rich in natural enzymes. However, these plants also contain enzyme inhibitors that prevent self-digestion. Without these inhibitors, the seeds, beans, and grains would ripen and decay before they could find the right location in which to germinate and grow. These foods have naturally extended shelf lives due to these inhibitors, but they can cause digestive difficulties when consumed because these inhibitors affect not only the enzymes contained in the plants, but also the enzymes produced by the digestive organs, thereby placing an extra burden on the pancreas. So if you eat raw seeds as snacks, be sure to take supplemental enzymes to reduce the stress on your digestive tract.

When seeds, beans and grains germinate, the inhibitors are deactivated. Cooking also deactivates many of the inhibitors, but experts differ as to whether it completely removes all of them.

When traveling, always have access to fresh fruits or vegetables. However, try to avoid highly acidic fruits like citrus and berries if you suffer from over acidity. Stop at a local market to stock up on high-enzyme foods like sprouts, carrots, celery, or papaya to snack on.

When eating in restaurants, concentrate on including as many salads, raw vegetables, and less acidic, more alkaline fruits such as melons and papayas. I also recommend you pack your own meal when traveling, particularly when you fly across time zones. For example, if you are flying from New York to Los Angeles and you arrive at your hotel at 9:00 p.m. (which for you is actually midnight), you will probably be too tired to go out for dinner—even if you have skipped the dinner served on the airplane and feel hungry.

Instead of raiding the room's refrigerator, which is filled with nutrient-poor, enzyme-deficient, highly acidic or acid-forming snacks like potato chips, peanuts, and colas, you'll have an energy-rich meal that you brought from home. Some raw, fresh vegetables, with a flavorful dressing or dip, a whole-grain muffin with some almond butter as a spread, and a piece of fruit (or a salad and fresh fruit ordered from room service) makes a great light supper that won't keep you up all night with indigestion. You'll wake up refreshed and ready to go in the morning.

Fermented Foods

Fermented foods are staples in the traditional cuisines of Europe, throughout the Mediterranean and Middle East, and in Asia, where the fermented tea *kombucha* is a common drink and fermented soy products such as soy sauce, shoyu, tamari, and tempeh are eaten every day. These cultured foods all contain living microorganisms that enhance the food's flavor, digestibility, and nutritional value, as well as acting as a preservative.

Many fermented foods are also rich sources of enzymes that enhance digestive function. Fermented foods include yogurt, sauerkraut, kefir (a beverage made from cow's milk), olives, pickles, beer, wine, vinegar, cheese, cottage cheese, and buttermilk. However, when these foods are commercially processed so that they have a longer shelf life, the enzymes can be destroyed. For the enzyme-rich, homemade version, it's best to shop in natural-food stores, which sometimes carry items such as freshly made sauerkraut, cured olives, and natural yogurt.

Combining Raw and Cooked Foods

It is not necessary to eat only raw foods to receive the digestive benefits of plant enzymes. Raw and cooked foods can be eaten in combination. A bowl of lentil soup and a carrot slaw provide legumes that are cooked (the lentils), coupled with living enzymes in the raw carrots. Poached salmon salad made with sliced onions and served on romaine lettuce is also a mix of both cooked and enzyme-rich raw ingredients.

People with weak digestive function may find when they eat mostly raw foods they can cause digestion symptoms like gas and bloating. Raw vegetables are made up of nonnutritive cellulose, which is tough, fibrous, and difficult for some individuals to digest. To make fibrous foods more easily digestible, it is important to chew them thoroughly.

For my patients with sensitive digestive systems, I recommend lightly steamed foods, easy-to-digest dishes like soups, and well-cooked grains along with side dishes of raw foods like salads. (As digestive function improves, my patients are usually able to tolerate more raw foods in their diets.) If you do enjoy salads and raw vegetables, it is fine to include these more and more in your meals as you restore your digestive function with enzyme-rich foods. However, I recommend making the transition slowly so that your body can adapt.

Step 2: Avoid Foods That Stress the Pancreas

As discussed earlier in this book, certain foods should be consumed minimally or not at all by people who are trying to restore their ability to produce pancreatic enzymes. These include wheat, red meat, and dairy products, which are all very hard to break down and require the body to produce large amounts of enzymes and other digestants like pepsin and hydrochloric acid. Such foods are also often high in saturated fats, sugars, and animal protein.

Some of these hard-to-digest foods are used in combinations to create dishes that are not only difficult to digest but may also be highly allergenic and acid-forming. The list includes mainstays of the standard American diet like pizza, barbecued ribs, cheese steaks, cheeseburgers, all fried foods including chicken, French fries and chips, donuts, pastries, ice cream, hot dogs, and chocolate.

For example, the pancreas must produce significant amounts of enzymes to digest a meal of steak, a fully dressed baked potato, buttered bread, wine, and chocolate cake for dessert. The meal is laden with saturated fats, red-meat protein, and sugar. Not only are the individual foods difficult to digest, but when mixed together they pose a formidable digestive task.

The difficulty that many people have digesting these foods is because you are often more tired after eating such a meal than you were before. In contrast, a light meal of bean soup, mixed green salad, and an undressed baked potato is full of vitamins, minerals, carbohydrates, and easy-to-digest vegetable-based protein. The pancreas is not overly stressed, and the digestive process proceeds efficiently, leaving you feeling energized and comfortable after eating.

Step 3: Drink Blenderized Drinks If Indicated

If you are a person with digestive problems or weak pancreatic function and suffer from a variety of inflammatory conditions, or even have a very serious health problem like cancer, one way to reduce the stress on the pancreas and help restore its functional capabilities is to drink blenderized meals.

Processing ingredients in a blender liquefies food, breaking all of its components into extremely small particles, and enhances (or replaces) the mechanical digestive step of chewing. The surface area of the food is dramatically increased, thereby eliminating one of the functions of pancreatic enzymes in the breakdown process and hence requiring less enzyme production. This takes an enormous amount of stress off of the pancreas and other digestive organs.

Liquefied food is partially predigested. It is absorbed and assimilated very easily, with minimal symptoms of incomplete or poor digestion such as bloating, gas, and food remaining in the digestive tract for long periods of time. The nutrients from the food are much more readily available when food is taken in blenderized form.

Foods such as vegetables, fruits, seeds, and nuts can be blenderized to make delicious shakes and drinks. Vegetables such as squash, turnips, yams, sweet potatoes, and potatoes can all be blenderized into purees. Thickened soups that are full of solids like beans and pieces of vegetables can be pureed and made easier to digest.

People with really weak digestive systems should consider blenderizing one to two meals per day while in the early stages of recovery. The third meal should consist of easily digestible solid food such as cooked salads, steamed vegetables, cooked grains, and meats like salmon or trout that tend to be softer and easier to digest than tougher, more fibrous meats like grilled steak. I have found that patients who substitute one or two blenderized meals per day have much more rapid healing and recovery times.

Blenderized drinks can be made from ingredients that are both enzyme-rich and more alkaline. Millions of Americans have both low digestive enzyme production and a tendency toward being overly acidic. Drinks such as these can provide therapeutic benefits for both conditions.

Liquefying the solid ingredients into a drink further reduces the workload of the pancreas and other digestive organs. These liquid meals can be extremely beneficial for conditions related to either over acidity or low enzyme production such as fatigue, brain fog, inflammatory conditions, autoimmune problems, and even cancer.

Any commercially available food processor or blender can be used; however, I have found that the Vitamix blenders (vitamix.com) are very powerful devices that can pulverize virtually any whole food into a liquid. This blender can emulsify raw or cooked foods and can be used for any combination of fruits, vegetables, seeds, nuts, liquids, or oils. In contrast, many juicers tend to extract the juice while discarding the nutrient-rich pulp.

Many athletes and others who require very high energy levels to perform in stressful or physically demanding jobs rely on one or two blenderized meals or snacks per day apart from their regular meals. Over the years, I have developed a number of drink recipes that provide protein, carbohydrates, and fats in an easily digestible form that can replace an entire solid meal.

Fruit Drinks

All of the ingredients in the following three recipes are readily available in health food stores, gourmet markets, and well-stocked supermarkets. I strongly recommend using organic ingredients whenever possible, since their nutrient content is higher than that of commercial-grade food. Although these delicious blenderized drinks can be used at any time of the day, many people prefer to have one for breakfast as these drinks can be made quickly and can easily be consumed in the car while commuting.

Raspberry Yogurt Smoothie   **Serves 1**

Raspberries are a great source of ellagic acid, an important antioxidant that helps to protect our cell membranes and other structures in the body from free radical damage. They also contain many other beneficial nutrients. The can be enjoyed freshly picked during the summer or frozen year around.

¼ cup nondairy yogurt; soy, almond, or coconut
(Goat milk yogurt may also be used.)
1 cup raspberries – fresh or frozen
1 banana
¾ cup rice milk
2 teaspoons protein powder
Sprinkle of Truvia (if desired)

Combine all ingredients in a blender. Puree until smooth and serve.

Peachy Flax Smoothie   Serves 1

If using frozen peaches, chopping the peaches beforehand will reduce the puree time in the blender.

½ cup orange juice
½ cup unsweetened rice milk
1 cup peaches – fresh or frozen
1 tablespoon rice protein powder
2 teaspoons ground flaxseed
1 banana, sliced

Combine all ingredients in a blender. Puree until smooth and serve.

Blueberry and Greens Shake   Serves 1

This drink is a powerhouse of nutrients! The chlorella and spirulina are powerful green foods. They are both available at health food stores. Now Foods makes a very good line of supplement products available at nowfoods.com

1 cup nondairy milk
⅔ cup blueberries – fresh or frozen
2 tablespoons protein powder
½ teaspoon chlorella
½ teaspoon spirulina
Sprinkle of Truvia (optional)

In a blender puree the nondairy milk and blueberries. Add rest of ingredients and blend well.

Individuals who have weak liver function in addition to diminished enzyme production may not be able to tolerate seeds, nuts, and their oils. If this is an issue for you, be cautious in making smoothies that contain any of these foods. See my book on detoxification if you need to restore your liver and detoxification capacity.

Vegetable Drinks

These three vegetable drinks are enzyme-rich "liquid salads," made by combining fresh vegetables and spring water in a blender or food processor that is capable of completely liquefying vegetables, such as the Vitamix blenders.

If you do not have such a powerful food processor, peel vegetables as directed. If you do, the peels can stay on if you like. The vegetables should be cut up into large pieces before putting them in the food processor.

Vegetable Drink No. 1   **Serves 1**

2 carrots, peeled
½ cup cooked beets
¼ cup parsley
1 stalk celery
2 cups spring or filtered water

Combine all the ingredients in a blender or food processor and run it on high speed for 60 to 90 seconds or until the drink is totally liquefied. Add more water if a thinner drink is desired. Drink immediately.

Vegetable Drink No. 2   Serves 1

⅓ cucumber, peeled
2 peeled garlic cloves
2 sprigs parsley
¼ large red bell pepper, seeded
½ cooked beet, outer layer scrubbed off
½ carrot, peeled
1 tablespoons olive oil
1 tablespoon maple syrup or rice bran syrup
½ teaspoon Bragg Liquid Aminos
2 cups spring or filtered water
4 or 5 ice cubes

Combine all the ingredients in a food processor or blender and run it on high speed for 60 to 90 seconds or until the drink is totally liquefied. Add more water if a thinner drink is desired. Drink immediately.

You can use this recipe as a base for experimenting with your favorite seasonal vegetables.

Vegetable Drink No. 3

Serves 1

2 carrots, peeled
½ cucumber, peeled
Few leaves of kale
1 stalk celery
1½-2 cups spring or filtered water

Combine all the ingredients in a blender or food processor and run it on high speed for 60 to 90 seconds or until the drink is totally liquefied. Add more water if a thinner drink is desired. Drink immediately.

If you suffer from over acidity or any inflammatory conditions, be sure to avoid adding such common hot, spicy, or acidic seasonings and flavorings as chili pepper, Tabasco sauce, black pepper, vinegar, citrus juices, Bloody Mary mix, and Worcestershire sauce, which can trigger symptoms of over acidity or inflammation. Many herbs can be safely used as flavoring agents. Naturally alkaline individuals can probably use most seasoning agents without ill effect unless they have a sensitivity to a particular one.

Step 4: Eat Pureed Foods If Indicated

Unlike blenderized drinks, pureed foods are usually cooked before being processed in a blender or food processor. While these are cooked foods and their enzymes have been deactivated, serving them in pureed form will significantly reduce stress on the digestive process, especially the pancreas. These recipes are especially helpful if you have digestive problems, weak pancreatic function, or a serious health problem.

Split Pea Soup Puree   **Serves 2 to 4**

1 cup dried split peas, picked over and rinsed
1 onion, chopped
2 carrots
4 cups spring or filtered water
¼ to ½ teaspoon sea salt or salt substitute

Combine the peas, onion, and carrots in a stockpot. Add water. Bring to a boil, then turn heat to low, and cover pot. Cook for 45 minutes. Add sea salt and continue cooking until peas are soft. Let soup cool, then puree in a blender or food processor until smooth.

Carrot Soup Puree   Serves 2 to 4

4 cups peeled and sliced carrots
2 cups diced onion
½ cup sweet red pepper
4 cups vegetable broth
1 cup rice or soy milk

Combine all the ingredients in a large stockpot. Cook for 30 minutes over medium heat or until carrots are tender. Let soup cool, then puree in a blender or food processor until smooth.

Butternut Squash Puree   Serves 2 to 4

1 large butternut squash, peeled and cubed
2 cups rice or soy milk
1 tablespoon rice bran syrup
ground nutmeg, allspice, or cinnamon to taste

Place the cut squash in a steamer and steam for 12 to 15 minutes or until very tender. While it is still hot, place the steamed squash in a blender or food processor. Add the nondairy milk and rice bran syrup and puree until smooth. Serve hot, with or without spices. This puree tastes like a rich dessert.

9

Take Supplemental Digestive Enzymes

There are a wide variety of plant- and animal-based digestive enzymes that you can take as supplements in addition to eating an enzyme-rich diet. In this chapter, I will discuss the two main types of supplemental enzymes available and how to use them for a number of conditions, such as digestive problems, sports injuries, surgical wounds, and respiratory infections.

I want to begin with a few important tips on the use of digestive enzymes, in general. It is important to remember that, when taken with a meal; supplemental enzymes will tend to be used in the digestive process. When taken between meals, on an empty stomach, the enzymes will instead be used by the body for their anti-inflammatory and cellular repair capabilities.

For those individuals who have both weak digestive function and other health conditions, the use of supplemental enzymes both with and apart from meals may be most appropriate.

Various forms of supplemental enzymes can be taken simultaneously. Many commercial preparations are, in fact, combinations of various enzymes. For example, you may take pancreatic enzymes, papain and bromelain, at the same time to enhance their therapeutic benefits with no adverse effects.

When you are customizing your program, it's helpful to know if your constitution tends to be more alkaline or more acidic. Most people in the United States are overly acidic. Many of these individuals also have low production of pancreatic enzymes. (If you want to know more about pH and how to support your acid/alkaline balance and health, see my book on this topic).

If you are overly acidic and enzyme deficient, avoid enzyme products that contain betaine or glutamic hydrochloric acid (HCl) as they may cause a burning sensation in the stomach or increase a tendency toward over acidity. If, on the other hand, you are one of the small number of individuals who have exceedingly good buffering capability, HCl supplementation combined with enzyme products may be beneficial.

The use of supplemental enzymes may cause side effects or detoxification symptoms because digestive enzymes, including pancreatic enzymes as well as bromelain and papain, are protein digestants. When taken supplementally, they will attack and begin to dissolve unhealthy tissue buildup in the body (which is their basis for use in alternative cancer treatments).

When they are used in large amounts or to excess, the breakdown process initiated by supplemental digestive enzymes can, on occasion, overwhelm the body's ability to remove these waste products. You may experience symptoms of detoxification, which are similar to those of a viral infection: a runny nose, flulike symptoms, unexplained fatigue, fever, skin eruptions, diarrhea, bad breath, muscle aches, or headaches.

This is your body telling you that you are eliminating waste products or cellular debris faster than your system can tolerate it. Side effects of excessive enzyme use include gas, bloating, and loose bowel movements. If these symptoms occur, reduce the dosage and/or frequency of supplementation until you reach a level that does not cause any symptoms.

You can also begin using procedures that promote healthy detoxification like liver flushes and coffee enemas which increase the body's ability to eliminate waste products before they reach levels that cause detoxification symptoms. I describe these techniques in detail in my book on detoxification.

Plant-Based Digestive Enzyme Supplements

I often recommend that my patients who have digestive complaints use supplemental plant-based digestive enzymes as part of their treatment program. These enzymes supplement those normally made by the stomach and pancreas. Like the digestive enzymes produced within our bodies, they help in the digestion of starches, protein, and fats. They are a convenient digestive aid for people who eat primarily cooked foods and for those eating their meals on the road, with limited access to fresh food.

The most readily available plant-based supplemental enzymes are bromelain and papain, which are sold in natural food stores and pharmacies. Besides assisting in the process of digestion, these enzymes are useful in the treatment of a variety of conditions, including trauma due to sports injuries, surgery, pancreatic insufficiency, respiratory tract infections, arthritis, angina, phlebitis painful menstruation, scleroderma, and prostatitis.

Bromelain

Bromelain refers to a family of enzymes extracted from the stem of the pineapple. It has been used over the centuries as a medicinal plant in tropical native cultures around the world and was isolated chemically over 100 years ago. In 1957, bromelain was introduced as a powerful therapeutic compound, used to assist digestion of protein and reduce inflammation.

Since then, over 200 scientific papers on its therapeutic applications have been published in the medical literature, ranging from treatment of the common cold to treatment of cancer. Following is a list of conditions that bromelain benefits, along with suggested dosages.

Digestion. As a digestive aid, bromelain can help to break down protein-rich foods such as red meat, dairy products, and wheat. Bromelain is most effective in improving digestion when it is taken with meals. Bromelain can also be used in the treatment of more severe digestive disorders such as gastric ulcers (an open sore or lesion of the mucous membrane of the stomach). An ulcer can produce symptoms of chronic pain, and if the erosion of the tissue is sufficient to cause bleeding, an ulcer can eventually be life threatening.

It is thought that the uptake of two compounds, glucosamine (a substance present in mucus) and radioactive sulfur, by the gastric mucosa may speed the healing of ulcers. In an animal study published in the *Hawaii Medical Journal*, researchers observed that bromelain increased the gastric uptake of glucose-amine by 30 to 90 percent, and of radioactive sulfur by 50 percent.

Bromelain supplementation is helpful when there is diminished pancreatic function and a reduced ability to produce pancreatic enzymes (pancreatic insufficiency). Unlike most digestive aids, bromelain remains active both in the stomach and in the small intestine, and has been shown in studies to be an adequate replacement for our own protein digesting enzymes, pepsin and trypsin.

A research study appearing in the *Journal of the Association of Physicians of India* evaluated the effectiveness of an enzyme preparation containing ox bile, bromelain, and pancreatin for the treatment of malabsorption syndrome, a condition in which soluble nutrients are poorly absorbed from the digestive tract, leading to digestive symptoms and weight loss. With the bromelain preparation, patients experienced needed weight gain and a greater sense of well-being. They also reported less pain, gas, and frequency of bowel movements.

Suggested Dosage: 500 to 1000 mg with a meal or immediately following meals.

Inflammation.　Nonsteroidal　anti-inflammatory drugs (NSAIDs) such as Ponstil and Naprosyn, are the most prescribed pharmaceutical agents in the United States, accounting for over 100 million prescriptions per year. In addition, tens of millions of individuals purchase anti-inflammatory medications over the counter, without a prescription.

While these medications are useful in reducing the symptoms of inflammation of many common conditions, from menstrual cramps to arthritis, by suppressing the production of all prostaglandins, they also suppress the beneficial anti-inflammatory ones. In addition, they have no effect on dissolving fibrin clots. Furthermore, long-term use of NSAIDs can lead to liver, kidney, and gastrointestinal side effects.

Unlike NSAIDs, bromelain acts as a natural aspirin without any of the undesirable side effects. Bromelain reduces inflammation in several ways. While aspirin inhibits the synthesis of all prostaglandins (hormone like chemicals produced within the intestinal tract, uterus, and other sites of the body), bromelain inhibits only the inflammatory ones, without affecting the anti-inflammatory ones.

Bromelain also interacts with fibrin, a tough, clot-like material made of protein that the body manufactures to seal off an injured area. When there is injury, caused by anything from a sports accident to bumping into the sharp corner of a desk, the blood vessels and capillaries in the injured area begin to dilate (expand) so the body's own healing substances can reach the area quickly.

At the same time, fluids force their way into the surrounding tissue, causing congestion and resulting in pressure, swelling, heat, and pain. Helper cells then begin to seal off the damaged area, creating fibrin clots made of protein.

In an effort to prevent the spread of bacteria and toxins generated by the injury, the fibrin also blocks blood and lymph vessels, which causes more swelling, a blockage of blood flow, and inflammation. The enzymes contained within bromelain help to reduce inflammation by digesting the fibrin clots.

In addition, supplemental bromelain helps to increase the oxygen level in injured tissue and stimulates the body's own natural enzymatic activity without suppressing the immune system, further accelerating the healing process.

Suggested Dosage: Bromelain supplements, in standard dosages of 500 mg taken two to four times per day, should be combined with bioflavonoids and vitamin C, as these enhance the action of bromelain. Recommended dosages are 500 to 1000 mg of bioflavonoids taken three times a day, and 1 g of vitamin C taken two or three times a day apart from meals.

Sports Injuries. Besides its usefulness in reducing inflammation due to illness, bromelain is also an effective treatment for a wide range of physical trauma. It is most typically used in the treatment of sports-related injuries. For example, if you strain your back playing golf on your day off, bromelain can speed your recovery and enable you to play again much sooner than you would otherwise expect.

In a research study reported in *Fortschritte Der Medizin*, fifty-nine patients (thirty-nine men and twenty women) with muscle strains, ligament tears, or contusions (a bruise or injury in which the skin is not broken) were given 500 mg of bromelain three times daily, thirty minutes before meals, for a period of one to three weeks.

Patients were evaluated for pain at rest and during motion, for swelling, and for tenderness. Patients also rated their own symptom levels. In every case, patients reported a reduction in all symptoms, with pain during motion and tenderness when touched showing the most improvement.

Various professions have a high risk of injury: law enforcement agents, firefighters, emergency workers, Red Cross volunteers, tree trimmers, employees in heavy industry, and members of the active military. The use of bromelain can be quite helpful in limiting the extent of any injury.

For example, bromelain has been used successfully in treating firefighters and police who have suffered injury in the line of duty. In Germany, prize fighters are directed to take enzymes before a fight to prevent the consequences of severe injuries. By using enzyme often, the usual forced inactivity during a two-month rest period after major injury can be reduced to several weeks.

My patient, Erica, was getting out of the car when she hit her foot on the curb and twisted her ankle. She told me that not only did her ankle hurt and swell but her entire body had stiffened up, too. I recommended a course of enzyme therapy, including bromelain, which helped to reduce the pain and swelling rapidly.

Patti, a long-time patient, complained that she was suffering from chronic low back pain and stiffness almost every morning when she would get out of bed. She tried a program of stretching which helped somewhat. I recommended a program of both a topical muscle relaxant and nutritional supplements including herbal muscle relaxants as well as bromelain. She was pleased to report that her back pain and stiffness had eased considerably.

Suggested Dosage: 500 to 1000 mg three to four times per day. Take between meals so that the bromelain is not used up in digesting food.

Most public institutions and private businesses keep aspirin and other NSAIDs available to employees to reduce the pain of minor injuries on the job. Having bromelain available also for these same purposes would help to speed up the healing process.

Surgical Wounds. Bromelain also speeds the healing of surgical wounds. An actress expressed her concern to me about how much time she would have to take off from work if she decided to undergo cosmetic surgery. I suggested a program of supplementation that included bromelain. The actress elected to have the surgery and immediately began my program. To her delight, she found that she healed much more rapidly than expected.

According to a study published in the *Journal of Oral Medicine*, a group of sixteen patients received bromelain therapy 4 times a day, beginning seventy-two hours prior to undergoing oral surgery. Twenty-four hours after surgery, 38 percent of the patients receiving bromelain had only mild pain or none at all, as compared with 13 percent of the untreated patients. Furthermore, one day after surgery, 75 percent of the treated patients had only mild inflammation or none at all, while only 19 percent of the untreated patients experienced a comparable reduction.

Bromelain is also effective in reducing the inflammation resulting from dental procedures such as root canals, tooth extractions, and dental surgery. It can also speed the healing of gum tissue, which can become irritated during dental procedures. For maximum effectiveness, it should be taken shortly before the procedure and immediately after it and continued until healing is complete.

Suggested Dosage: Begin the use of enzymes one to two days prior to the dental or surgical procedure and continue until the healing is complete — 500 to 1000 mg four times per day apart from meals.

Respiratory Tract Infections. Nasal congestion due to respiratory tract infections is a nuisance, hampering almost any activity. There is scientific evidence that bromelain can be very useful in the treatment of upper respiratory problems that generate mucus. Bromelain decreases the volume and viscosity of mucus so that it can be more easily cleared from the respiratory tract.

This was shown in a study published in *Drugs Under Experimental and Clinical Research*. The volunteers included seventy men and fifty-four women; aged 35 to 75, hospitalized with lung diseases such as chronic bronchitis, pneumonia, and pulmonary abscess.

Patients were randomly given one of three therapies: amoxicillin plus 80 mg of bromelain, amoxicillin plus indomethacin, or amoxicillin alone, every eight hours, for at least eight days or as needed. The sputum (substance expelled by coughing or clearing the throat) of the patients was then analyzed for viscosity.

The results of this study showed that bromelain significantly increased the fluidity of mucus. There was also evidence that bromelain combined with drug therapy enhanced the absorption of the amoxicillin.

My patient, Carol, had been suffering from recurrent bronchial infections and colds that caused her to miss work as often as once or twice a month. She suffered frequently from nasal congestion and coughing, despite the use of medication prescribed by her physician. I recommended that she begin taking bromelain, along with other powerful supplements. She was thrilled to report that her chest was much clearer and that her episodes of colds and bronchitis had become much less frequent.

Suggested Dosage: 500 to 1000 mg four to six times per day. Take both with and apart from meals.

Using Bromelain with Antibiotics. Several studies in the scientific literature document the effectiveness of bromelain in enhancing the action of antibiotics. In one research study, published in *Experimental Medicine & Surgery*, fifty-three hospitalized patients were given combined antibiotic and bromelain therapy to treat such potentially life-threatening diseases as pneumonia, bronchitis, thrombophlebitis, pyelonephritis, and rectal abscesses. Twenty-three of these patients had been unsuccessfully treated with antibiotic therapy alone. Of these, twenty-two responded favorably to the combined therapy.

Researchers also compared the length of stay for patients taking antibiotics alone or the combined therapy. Patients with pneumonia or bronchitis who were treated with antibiotics alone remained in the hospital for an average of ten days, as compared with those who also received enzyme therapy, who were able to leave the hospital after only six days.

Another study, published in the journal *Headache*, looked at the use of bromelain in combination with antibiotics for the treatment of acute sinusitis. Forty-eight patients were placed on standard therapy, which included antihistamines and analgesic agents, along with antibiotics, if indicated. Twenty-three patients received bromelain four times daily, while the remaining twenty-five received a placebo. Of the patients receiving bromelain, eighty-seven percent had complete resolution of nasal mucosal inflammation, compared with only fifty-two percent in the placebo group.

The next time you come down with an acute infection and your doctor writes you a prescription for antibiotics, be sure to supplement that medication with bromelain. Along with rest, supplementing with bromelain will help you return to your usual activities much more quickly.

Heart Disease. Patients with cardiovascular disease may benefit from taking digestive enzymes since bromelain can help to reduce platelet aggregation or clumping. Platelets are a component of the blood that, when they clump, can increase the risk of heart attack and stroke. Use of digestive enzymes can reduce this tendency of platelets to be sticky.

The first conclusive evidence that bromelain prevents clumping of blood platelets (aggregation) was reported in the journal *Experientia*. Twenty volunteers with a history of heart attack or stroke, or with high platelet aggregation values, were given bromelain. In seventeen of the subjects, bromelain decreased aggregation of blood platelets. Oral pancreatic digestive enzyme preparations are also regularly used in Europe to help dissolve clots in the veins. Numerous studies confirm their usefulness in dissolving small clots (microthrombi), which helps to prevent the development of large clots that may eventually trigger a vascular accident.

Suggested Dosage: 500 to 1000 mg three to four times a day apart from meals.

Factors that can Inactivate Bromelain. Certain metallic compounds are known to render bromelain inactive, including copper and iron, which are found naturally in many foods, and the heavy metals lead, mercury, and cadmium, which are sometimes present as toxic pollutants in fish and other foods. Heavy metal contamination can also be found in poor-quality, commercial-grade foods. Buying the highest quality organically grown foods will help you to avoid these enzyme inhibitors.

When shopping for a bromelain supplement, avoid those that combine the bromelain with copper or iron in the same tablet or capsule. Look for bromelain combined with magnesium or cysteine, bromelain activators that enhance its therapeutic effect. The quality of bromelain is expressed in gelatin-digesting units (g.d.u.). The higher the g.d.u., the higher the grade of bromelain and its activity. Keep in mind that bromelain is not heat stable, so supplements need to be stored in a cool place.

Papain

Papain is the enzyme derived from papayas. Best known as a meat tenderizer, it can also be used as a powerful digestant of protein either by itself or combined with bromelain and other digestive enzymes. Research has found that papain has many other clinical applications, such as aiding in recovery from injuries and surgery, and treating a number of inflammatory conditions such as gluten intolerance.

Digestive Problems. Papain has been found to be helpful for digestive problems such as gluten intolerance. Gluten is the protein found in wheat; gluten intolerance can cause intestinal inflammation, bloating, cramping, and gas.

An interesting case study, published in *The Lancet*, documented the use of papain in the treatment of gluten intolerance. The authors reported that the patient studied was first put on a gluten-free diet, which produced symptom relief and some weight gain. However, the patient's steatorrhea (fatty stools) continued. He was then treated with papain. After four weeks of therapy, his intestinal absorption returned to normal. Subsequently, when the patient reintroduced gluten-containing foods in his diet, he experienced no further symptoms of an intolerance to gluten.

Suggested Dosage: 200 to 300 mg with a meal or immediately following meals, upon rising, and before bedtime.

Traumatic Injuries. A variety of traumatic injuries, such as those resulting from playing sports, can be aided by the use of papain. A two-year study, published in *Current Therapeutic Research*, followed the recovery time of 125 members of athletic teams, predominantly football, who received mild to moderate injuries during games or practice. The players were monitored for swelling, pain, and skin discoloration due to bleeding within tissues (ecchymosis).

Of the sixty-five patients treated with papain (Carica papaya), nearly 70 percent showed a better than expected response to the therapy. Only 20 percent of the sixty untreated patients in the study had comparable recovery. The anti-inflammatory benefits of the papain allowed the players to return to their athletic activities sooner than anticipated.

Suggested Dosage: 200 mg four times per day apart from meals.

Inflammatory Conditions. Along with bromelain, papain is also useful in the treatment of inflammatory conditions that affect our cells and tissues, such as respiratory infections like colds, flus, bronchitis, arthritis, and thyroiditis.

Suggested Dosage: 200 to 300 mg with a meal or immediately following meals, upon rising, and before bedtime.

Minor Surgery and Dental Procedures. Millions of individuals annually undergo minor surgery and dental procedures such as tooth extractions and root canals. While these procedures are usually not life threatening, they can cause significant pain and discomfort. The use of papain can reduce these uncomfortable symptoms and help speed up the healing process.

Papain, like bromelain, is also an effective treatment for postoperative complications after oral surgery — specifically, after the removal of impacted molars, according to a study published in the *Journal of the American Dental Association.* A group of 129 patients were given either papase or prednisolone (a synthetic form of the anti-inflammatory hormone cortisol) or were left untreated. Patients were given therapy postoperatively and evaluated for pain, edema (water retention in tissue), and trismus (the postsurgical spasm of the muscles of chewing).

While no significant differences were found for edema between the treated and untreated groups, both papase and prednisolone were found to be effective at reducing trismus and pain. An added benefit of the natural enzyme therapy is that there are virtually no side effects associated with its use.

Suggested Dosage: 200 mg four times per day apart from meals.

Organic Green Papaya

Aside from papain, ground dried organic green papaya is also very high in its digestive enzyme content. This can be found in natural food stores or by mail order. Take to 1 to 3 tsp. with meals as a digestive aid and natural anti-inflammatory.

Side Effects of Plant Enzymes

While plant enzymes are not known to cause any serious side effects, they may cause increased intestinal gas. Gradually increasing your dosage can improve your tolerance and reduce the likelihood of gas. Plant enzymes should be avoided, as should most supplements, by pregnant women and people with any kind of bleeding disorder.

Pancreatic Enzymes Derived from Animal Sources

Although commercial preparations of supplemental pancreatic enzymes are actually derived from the pancreas of animals, particularly cows and pigs, these enzymes are similar to those found in the human body.

Pancreatic enzyme products are unique because they are able to break down all three basic food substances found in our diets: carbohydrates, proteins, and fats. In other words, they contain protein digesting (proteolytic), fat digesting (lipolytic), and starch and sugar digesting (glycolytic) capability.

Pancreatic enzymes, whether produced within the body or taken as supplements, are necessary for normal digestive function. They are also powerful anti-inflammatory and anticlotting agents. Their action occurs at the tissue level in various parts of the body, including muscle and epidermal (skin) tissue.

Supplemental pancreatic enzymes can also improve digestion, reducing the workload on the body's own pancreatic enzymes, and facilitate healing from sports injuries or other traumas or after surgery. Following is a list of health conditions benefited by pancreatic enzymes and the suggested dosages for the enzymes. While these can be taken alone, they are frequently combined in nutritional supplement products with plant-based digestive enzymes.

Digestive Problems. Pancreatic enzymes are helpful in supporting pancreatic insufficiency and digestive symptoms such as gas and bloating.

Suggested Dosage: One to two 300 to 500 mg tablets with meals or directly following meals. Commercial products may vary between 100 and 500 mg, with many products in the 300 to 500 mg range.

Traumatic Injuries. Numerous studies attest to the remarkable ability of these enzymes to speed recovery time and reduce the symptoms of sports injuries. According to a study in *The Practitioner*, enzymes wcrc found to be of great benefit when used by English football (soccer) associations to treat soft tissue injury and damage to ligaments.

Many decades ago, during thc 1964–65 season, the researchers gave enzymes for the first time ever to twenty-eight first-team players and kept track of their injuries. Up to that time, athletes were treated with the usual medical procedures as well as graded exercises, massage, and careful supervision.

The researchers found that prior to enzyme therapy athletes on the teams had lost an average of fifteen days of play during the preceding season. However, with enzyme therapy, the same players lost an average of only eleven days. In a further study, 131 soccer players who were not taking enzymes missed games because of injury, while only 90 athletes who were taking enzymes were unable to play.

As with soccer, karate injuries can occur in every area of the body. In an interesting study, a variety of injuries responded quite rapidly to enzyme treatment. Ten karate fighters of both sexes were treated with enzyme tablets before competition, while a second group received no enzymes.

During play, all the athletes had injuries comparable in severity. In the athletes treated with enzymes, hematomas (a swelling or mass of blood confined to a tissue and caused by a break in a blood vessel) disappeared within six and a half days, compared with nearly sixteen days in the untreated group. Swelling subsided after approximately four days in the treated group, compared with nearly ten days in the untreated group.

Restriction of movement resolved after five days in the group treated with enzymes, compared with over twelve and a half days in the untreated group. In addition, inflammatory symptoms resolved rapidly, taking only four days to subside in the treated group, compared with ten and a half days in the players not taking enzymes.

Annie, one of my patients, began to take advantage of the benefits of enzymes several years ago when she entered one of the numerous golf tournaments held at her country club. Usually, when a tournament lasted more than one day, she would notice stiffness or soreness on the second day. But when she began to use enzymes prophylactically, the second day of play felt as comfortable as the first. The remarkable ability of enzymes to heal or actually prevent the stiffness or soreness incurred by the occasional or weekend athlete have made participating in these events much more enjoyable.

Suggested Dosage: One to two 300 to 500 mg tablets, four times a day, apart from meals.

Many weekend warriors and people who like to take sports-oriented vacations can benefit from the use of supplemental pancreatic enzymes. If you plan to have several days of vigorous activity, skiing for the weekend or spending a week at a golf or tennis camp, be sure to supplement your diet with pancreatic enzymes during this period. Enzymes will minimize the stiffness and soreness you may feel after your first day's workout and enzymes can provide prophylactic treatment of strains or injuries that may occur.

Besides sports injuries, pancreatic enzymes can also be an important part of a healing regimen for injuries sustained on the job and accidents in general. Enzymes can be used to shorten employee time away from the office and may help to reduce disability. They should be a staple of on-site nursing facilities for companies whose employees have a higher risk of injury, such as construction workers and people working in assembly plants. Enzyme therapy can be a money-saving management strategy.

Repetitive Stress Injuries. People who are required to use their hands for their work, such as computer programmers and casino dealers, may develop inflammation in the forearm, or tenosynovitis, caused by repetitive motion. In this ailment, the tissues around tendons (synovial sheaths) become inflamed. A person with this disease cannot use their hands in fine, delicate movements.

A study appearing in *Clinical Medicine* examined the effect of proteolytic-enzyme therapy in treating tenosynovitis. Sixty men who worked in South Africa as cane cutters (a type of work requiring repetitive movements over many hours and days) were divided into two groups. Twenty-eight of the volunteers were given enzyme therapy four times a day for five days, and their swelling, pain, and range of arm movement monitored. These disabling symptoms resolved far more rapidly in the treated group than for those workers not receiving enzymes.

Suggested Dosage: One to two 300 to 500 mg tablets, four times a day, apart from meals.

Autoimmune Disease. As discussed in chapter 5, pancreatic enzymes can reduce levels of circulating immune complexes (CIC's). These are formed when large protein molecules, only partially digested in the small intestine, are absorbed into the bloodstream. The immune system treats these molecules as invaders. Antibodies couple with them and CICs are formed. CICs are found in such autoimmune diseases as thyroiditis, Crohn's disease, and rheumatoid arthritis.

German researchers found that a reduction in levels of CICs in patients with rheumatoid arthritis was associated with an improvement in health. In a study published in *Zeitschrift für Rheumatologie*, forty-two patients with rheumatoid arthritis were given the pancreatic enzyme preparation Wobenzym for a period of six weeks.

During this time, researchers monitored the patients both for changes in their symptoms and for levels of CICs. At the end of the test period, over 60 percent of the patients had a reduction in their symptoms, and these improvements were positively correlated with a decrease in levels of CICs.

Suggested Dosage: One to two 300 to 500 mg tablets, four times a day, apart from meals.

Surgery. Pancreatic enzymes can benefit surgical patients and patients experiencing delayed healing. One of the biggest concerns that my patients facing surgery voice is their fear of getting behind in their work if they do not recover rapidly.

This is a particular concern for people who are self-employed and cannot afford much time away from work since they have no disability insurance to fall back on. The use of pancreatic enzymes can speed up the surgical healing process and help people return to work and productive activity much more rapidly.

A powerful pancreatic enzyme product produced in Germany has been tested in several clinical trials in the treatment of surgery patients. One such study, presented at the FIMS World Congress of Sports Medicine, was conducted by researchers at a surgical clinic in Wiesbaden. They assessed the effect of enzyme treatment on recovery time after knee surgery.

Using eighty volunteers, the researchers treated half of the patients with enzymes. Those receiving enzymes regained mobility more rapidly than the untreated patients, and had less postoperative edema (retention of fluid in the tissues). In a second study, the same researchers tested the effects of enzyme treatment given preoperatively on 120 patients awaiting surgical treatment of fractures. On the day of surgery, those patients receiving enzymes had far less edema and less pain than the untreated patients.

In another study, published in *Clinical Medicine*, digestive enzymes were shown to be effective for treatment of traumatic swelling due to oral and maxillofacial surgery. The enzyme chymotrypsin was given, four times daily, to twenty-two patients having maxillofacial (involving the jawbone) and routine oral surgery. Treatment was started at the time of surgery or immediately afterward. The actual swelling experienced by the patients after twenty-four hours was about one-third of that normally anticipated. In addition, the thirteen patients with maxillofacial injuries evidenced rapid, and in some cases, dramatic recovery.

Suggested Dosage: Begin taking one 300 to 500 mg tablet one to two days before the surgery and continue until healing is complete. Take apart from meals.

Childbirth. Pancreatic enzymes can be very useful in obstetric care for women giving birth. Obstetricians will often perform an episiotomy, a small incision in the perineum made to avoid tearing of the tissues as the baby leaves the birth canal. The use of supplemental pancreatic enzymes can reduce the pain and edema associated with the procedure.

In a double-blind study published in the *American Journal of Obstetrics and Gynecology*, of 204 episiotomy patients, 111 received proteolytic-enzyme treatment. The volunteers were evaluated for pain when moving, sitting, and at rest, plus edema and ecchymosis (skin discoloration due to bleeding within tissues). Enzymes were given as patients were admitted to the labor room and were continued for five days postpartum. The researchers noted that the enzyme treatment reduced edema during the three days after childbirth, when it is usually greatest, and that pain and ecchymosis were also reduced.

Suggested Dosage: One to two 300 to 500 mg tablets, four times a day, apart from meals.

Pancreatitis. Pancreatic enzymes are used as replacement therapy in the treatment of chronic pancreatitis, a severe inflammatory condition, often caused by excessive alcohol use, which results in destruction of the structure as well as the enzyme producing capability of the pancreas.

In a study appearing in the *New England Journal of Medicine*, researchers monitored six patients with advanced pancreatic insufficiency (a condition in which the pancreas is no longer able to produce the requisite amount of enzymes needed for healthy digestive function).

The patients were assessed for their response to treatment with pancreatin taken with cimetidine (a drug that decreases secretion of gastric acid during both the day and night), pancreatin taken alone, cimetidine taken alone, and no medication at all.

With the combination of pancreatin and cimetidine, the digestive enzymes trypsin and lipase were restored after meals to significantly higher levels than with the medication alone. Further, this was the only treatment that fully prevented four of the six patients from having bowel movements that contained abnormally high levels of fat, which would normally be absorbed into the body. Pancreatin also allowed for better fat absorption when taken alone, as compared with neutralizing antacids.

Pancreatic enzymes have also been used in the treatment of a wide range of other inflammatory health problems, including sinusitis, hay fever, rheumatoid arthritis, and cystic fibrosis.

Suggested Dosage: One to two 300 to 500 mg tablets four times a day, apart from meals to promote healing. Also consider using with meals to support better digestive function.

Cancer. Pancreatic enzymes have also been used in the treatment of cancer. As mentioned earlier in this book, the Scottish embryologist John Beard initiated the research on this, and certain modern alternative cancer treatment specialists have applied his theories, incorporating the aggressive use of pancreatic enzymes in their own cancer treatment programs.

The most prominent of these specialists is Nicholas Gonzalez, who was trained as an immunologist. Gonzalez uses a protocol based on the work of William Donald Kelley. A dentist by training, Kelley was diagnosed with probable pancreatic cancer and cured himself by taking high doses of pancreatic enzymes. He also underwent an extensive liver detoxification program through the use of coffee enemas, as well as tailoring his diet to his metabolic type. Kelley subsequently treated many patients for a variety of cancers using these basic principles.

While in medical school, Gonzalez had begun an informal study of the effectiveness of taking a nutritional approach to treating cancer. A friend told him about Kelley's work. Gonzalez met with Kelley and was so impressed that he eventually began a five-year research project under the direction of Robert Good, former president of the Memorial Sloan Kettering Institute. Gonzalez found Kelley's patient records to be meticulous, and he subjected Kelley's results to rigorous analysis.

Gonzalez also searched out many of the patients Kelley had treated and was able to meet and/or talk with them firsthand. Gonzalez was able to confirm that Kelley's patients with pancreatic cancer, a cancer with negligible survival rates, had a remarkable survival rate using Kelley's protocols.

Consequently, Gonzalez developed a protocol based on the Kelley program, and in 1989, began using this protocol with patients. In 1997, he completed a study in cooperation with the National Cancer Institute, in which he used enzymes to treat twelve patients with pancreatic cancer. The study began in December 1993, with a patient who had cancer that was inoperable. By 1997, of the twelve patients, seven were still alive and doing well, two who had not been fully compliant had died, and three who had been compliant also died.

Current medical treatments for pancreatic cancer offer a survival time of one year or less for most patients. All of the patients in the study lived longer than had been predicted. Further, one reason that some of the patients did not survive is that they entered the program near death, or with cancers in a very advanced stage.

Dr. Gonzalez's program includes a specific diet and aggressive use of nutritional supplements, as well as both digestive enzyme and pancreatic enzyme therapy. Detoxification is also a critical part of the treatment to aid the body in eliminating the waste products and toxins that result from the breakdown of tumors.

Gonzalez speculates that some of the poor survival rates of current treatment modalities result from the inability of the patient to eliminate the breakdown products from the tumors. Gonzalez recommends coffee enemas to avoid any toxic buildup in the body,

The German enzyme product Wobenzym, which is available in the United States, is used in complementary cancer therapy. It is recommended that the pancreatic enzymes be taken at other than mealtimes in order to maintain their tumor-destroying effects. The enzymes are often administered on a set schedule at intervals throughout the day and night. Obviously, making sure to wake up in the middle of the night to take these can be a nuisance. However, practitioners who prescribe enzymes have found them to be quite helpful in the treatment of a variety of tumors. Thus, disrupting one's sleep may be worthwhile, given the potential benefits.

If cancer is of specific concern, please contact an appropriate physician in your area. See the appendix for names, addresses, and phone numbers for associations of physicians practicing complementary medicine.

How to Use Pancreatic Enzymes

Pancreatic enzyme products are available in natural food stores and are sold as tablets or capsules that can vary greatly in size of dose and potency. The potency is indicated by a notation on the label, which is usually a number followed by an X, for instance, 4X or 10X.

These have been strictly defined by the United States Pharmacopoeia (USP). In a 1X pancreatic-enzyme product (pancreatin), each milligram must contain at least 25 USP units of amylase activity, at least 25 USP units of protease activity, and at least 2.0 USP units of lipase activity.

Any pancreatic enzyme of higher potency is noted with a whole number greater than 1 to indicate the degree of its greater strength. For example, a pancreatic extract, full-strength and undiluted, that is eight times stronger than the USP standard would be labeled 8X USP. Full-strength products are generally preferred, as lower-potency pancreatic products may be diluted with substances such as lactose, galactose, and salt.

Pancreatic enzymes are dispensed as powders, capsules, granules, and tablets, the last two available in enteric-coated forms (this means that they don't break down in the stomach). Pancreatic enzyme supplements with enteric coating may have an advantage because the protective coating allows the pH-sensitive enzymes to pass through the hostile acidic environment of the stomach without being destroyed. Enteric-coated tablets are more likely to reach the small intestine intact, where they are normally used by the body to assist in the breakdown and digestion of foods.

Suggested Dosage: A standard dosage of pancreatic enzymes is one to two tablets, taken with meals if they are meant to be used as a digestive aid. Follow the instructions on the bottle. If a stronger treatment is needed, buy a more potent enzyme product.

If pancreatic enzymes are used to treat an anti-inflammatory disease such as rheumatoid arthritis, an accepted dosage is 300 to 1000 mg of high-potency pancreatic enzymes, taken three to four times a day, apart from meals.

When pancreatic enzymes are used in this manner, the supplements need to be taken at least four times a day, because the enzymes are only active in the body for a maximum of five hours.

It is essential that pancreatic enzymes be taken when the stomach is empty, preferably one-half to one hour before meals, because a considerable amount of the enzymes' ability to digest protein is lost in the acid environment of the stomach.

Some enzyme products are enteric-coated, that is, buffered by chemicals like sodium bicarbonate so they will not be attacked by gastric acid or pepsin in the stomach. However, numerous studies have found these to be no more effective, and in some cases, less effective, than uncoated enzymes.

Side Effects of Pancreatic Enzymes

It is well documented in scientific research studies that pancreatic enzymes are remarkably free of side effects. However, an excess dosage of these enzymes may cause diarrhea, especially in older patients, and bowel tolerance needs to be monitored. The need for these enzymes diminishes as health returns, and dosages can then be slowly decreased.

10

Use Other Natural Anti-Inflammatory Agents

For the treatment of acute and chronic inflammatory conditions, there are a number of natural anti-inflammatory agents that can be used in combination with digestive enzymes for even better results. These agents are available in most natural food stores as nutritional supplements. A number of research studies attest to their ability to speed recovery time for many ailments. Because they have minimal or no side effects, they offer a safe way to treat a wide variety of inflammatory conditions.

MSM

Methylsulfonylmethane (MSM) is one of the most powerful anti-inflammatories derived from natural foods. MSM is a nontoxic, physiologically active sulfur compound that is a breakdown product of DMSO (dimethyl oxide).

DMSO was originally used in the United States only as an industrial solvent. It is now recognized as having significant medical applications and is an FDA-approved treatment for interstitial cystitis, an inflammatory bladder ailment. DMSO is also used extensively by veterinarians for the treatment of a wide variety of inflammatory conditions in animals.

A person taking DMSO may experience side effects such as dry skin and a fishy body odor. MSM is preferable as a therapeutic agent as it is odorless and virtually tasteless and causes no aftertaste when taken by mouth.

MSM functions as the flexible bond between proteins. When a cell dies, a new cell takes its place. Without the needed amount of MSM, cells and tissues lose their flexibility, and problems develop within the lungs and other parts of the body. In its role as an anti-inflammatory agent, MSM may facilitate the production of certain enzymes needed to counteract inflammation. As an anti-parasitic, MSM is thought to block binding sites for parasites in the intestinal and urogenital tracts.

MSM is a component of all normal diets in verte-brates, but seems to be required in higher amounts than a typical diet provides. Cow's milk is a primary source of MSM for humans. However, since many people are allergic to or intolerant of cow's milk, they are unable to obtain MSM from this source. Since the body's levels of MSM tend to diminish with age, it is necessary to use supplemental sources after midlife to maintain essential tissue support.

Stanley W. Jacobs, a professor of surgery at the medical school of the University of Oregon, has conducted the primary research on MSM. According to an article by Jacobs and Herschler published in the *Annals of the New York Academy of Sciences*, MSM has been shown to reduce the tendency toward food allergies and allowed food-sensitive individuals to eat foods that they would normally not have been able to tolerate.

It also decreases the sensitivity to certain drugs such as anti-arthritic agents and antibiotics. Finally, MSM can function as an antacid and can be used for the treatment of constipation as well as parasitic and fungal infections. Dr. Jacobs has also found MSM to have anti-inflammatory and analgesic (pain-relieving) benefits when used to treat health problems such as interstitial cystitis, scleroderma, and systemic lupus erythematosus.

Supplemental MSM can also be used prophylactically before any strenuous physical activity. According to an article published in the newsletter of the *American Holistic Medical Association*, runners have found MSM to be of benefit when taken before a race to prevent joint pain, muscle soreness, and fatigue. The article also mentions that in veterinary medicine, MSM has been given to racehorses for many years to prevent them from having symptoms of physical stress after running a race.

Suggested Dosage: 250 to 750 mg of MSM granules taken three times per day in divided doses with meals or before undertaking a strenuous activity.

Colloidal Silver

Reducing or eliminating infection, either bacterial or viral, will eliminate one of the major causes of inflammation. Inflammation results from the body's immune response as it tries to destroy the bacteria or virus. Further inflammation results from the highly acidic waste products eliminated by the bacteria or viruses.

For centuries, silver has been known to be an effective antibacterial substance. In ancient civilizations, water was stored in silver vessels to keep bacteria from growing in it, and people in the nineteenth century often put a silver dollar in milk to retard spoilage. In the early twentieth century, colloidal silver was shown to be a very effective antibiotic and antiviral substance for eliminating or preventing many minor internal and external infections. Today it is recognized that colloidal silver is effective against over 650 disease-causing organisms.

A colloid is a substance that consists of extremely fine particles suspended in another medium such as water. Colloidal silver is, therefore, submicroscopic clusters of pure metallic silver suspended in distilled water. It is created by electrolysis.

In this process, an electrical current is passed between two poles, one of which is pure silver. The electric current breaks off microscopic pieces of the silver (a particle size of 0.0001 micron), and these particles stay suspended in the water due to their electrical charge. The particles are measured in parts per million (ppm); most commercially available products range from 5 to 500 ppm.

Studies show that many viruses, bacteria, and fungi are rendered ineffective (in vitro) in three to four minutes after exposure to colloidal silver. Although the exact mechanism of action is not known, it appears that the silver affects enzymes in the cells of the bacteria, inhibiting their replication.

Colloidal silver is nontoxic at prescribed doses. It is tasteless and odorless and can be taken orally or applied to the skin by either spraying it on or using it in a salve form. It does not irritate the eyes, and when applied to wounds or scrapes, it does not sting.

Even though it is a powerful antibiotic, when taken in prescribed doses, it does not destroy the "friendly" bacteria in the intestinal tract. Unlike pharmaceutical antibiotics, colloidal silver never permits strain-resistant pathogens to develop. Colloidal silver can be used wherever and whenever an antibacterial or antiviral agent is indicated. It can be used both to treat existing conditions and as a preventive agent.

Recent research indicates that many more health conditions may be caused by bacteria than had been previously thought. For example, peptic ulcers and rheumatoid arthritis are now thought to be caused, in part, by bacteria.

In a study published in an issue of the *Journal of the American Medical Association*, researchers found support that bacterial infections could be a cause of heart disease, the nation's number one killer. They found that people who have taken certain antibiotics may reduce their risk of heart disease — in effect, by containing or eliminating the causative strain of bacteria.

Colloidal silver can be purchased at health food stores or made at home using inexpensive battery-powered electrolysis units. It is available in dropper bottles in strengths varying from 5 to 500 ppm. (Lower strengths of 5 to 10 ppm are more optimal.)

When taking it orally, you should allow it to remain in the mouth for thirty to sixty seconds so that the microscopic particles of pure silver can be absorbed through the mucosal lining, bypassing the digestive tract. When using it on the skin, transfer the colloidal silver solution to a spray bottle and spray it on the affected area.

Suggested Dosage: Take two dropperfuls every two to four hours for an acute infection, decreasing to every 6-8 hours as symptoms begin to resolve.

Colostrum

Colostrum is the first milk produced by all mammals after delivery of the newborn. While maternal milk provides important nutrients that are needed for growth and development, colostrum is crucial to the newborn's health since it enhances immunity.

Studies have shown that breast-fed human infants have better resistance to a variety of diseases, including respiratory illnesses, than bottle-fed ones. This is because colostrum contains cytokines and other low molecular weight protein compounds that act as biologic response modulators. These substances have profound anti-inflammatory and immunity enhancing effects.

In one study published in the *British Medical Journal*, samples of human colostrum were examined and all contained respiratory virus neutralizing benefits. Immunoglobulin IgA was found in 18 out of 21 samples. IgA is known to confer protection against upper respiratory infections. This same study also found that breast feeding conferred significant protection against respiratory illness in infants. Far fewer breast fed infants were admitted to a hospital with severe respiratory illness versus non breast fed infants.

In another research study published in *Pediatrics*, infants in Bangladesh were followed from birth to twelve months of age. Exclusive breastfeeding in these infants was found to have significant protection against death from acute respiratory illnesses as well as death from diarrhea.

This enhanced immunity is one reason why breast feeding is so beneficial for infants. I recommend that every mother breast feed her child until at least one year of age, if at all possible. I have seen a number of infants below the age of a year and a half with frequent respiratory infections. Often, these infants have been fed commercial formulas instead of breast milk, either from birth or because the mother discontinued breast feeding after a month or two. Infants who have food allergies to dairy and other common foods are at particular risk when not breast fed.

Adults can benefit, too, from colostrum supplementation. In a research study published in the *European Journal of Nutrition*, bovine colostrum appeared to prevent upper respiratory infections in adult men, again probably through increasing immunoglobulins, specifically salivary IgA.

A number of research studies have also found colostrum to be helpful in the treatment of diseases such as rheumatoid arthritis, endometriosis, prostatitis, gluten intolerance, allergies, colds, and herpes simplex infection. While human colostrum is not readily available and can be very expensive, concentrated derivatives of bovine colostrum are available in health food stores or the Internet. Bovine colostrum supplements are available in either a spray or a chewable enzyme.

Suggested Dosage: Use as a spray or lozenge twice a day. The product is usually held in the mouth for a minute or two to promote absorption through the mucosal lining. It is also available as capsules. Treatment times vary between two weeks and six months.

Alkalinizing Agents

Maintaining the cells and tissues of the body in their healthy, slightly alkaline state helps to prevent inflammation. In contrast, over acidity can promote the onset of painful and disabling inflammatory conditions as diverse as colds, sinusitis, rheumatoid arthritis, and interstitial cystitis.

The use of alkalinizing agents like sodium and potassium bicarbonate or even sodium bicarbonate alone (baking soda in ½ to 1 teaspoon dosages taken upon arising and before going to bed at night) in combination with digestive enzymes and other natural anti-inflammatory supplements can be extremely helpful in healing many different types of inflammatory conditions.

Quercetin

Quercetin, a natural substance, is a member of the flavonoid family. Flavonoids are substances found in nature in many plants that have anti-inflammatory, anti-allergenic, anti-viral, anti-carcinogenic, and anti-microbial effects. Flavonoids are also potent free radical scavengers, antioxidants, and metal chelators, which bind to iron and copper and help eliminate them from the body.

Quercetin belongs to a subgroup of flavonoids called flavones and flavonols (commonly called bioflavonoids in products available in natural-food stores). Quercetin is naturally available in high amounts in plants such as onions. In experimental studies, quercetin displays the highest degree of activity of any flavonoid compound and is known to be highly effective in lowering inflammation.

Quercetin helps to maintain the strength of small blood vessels and to reduce vascular fragility. This counteracts the tendency toward bleeding problems and bruising, as well as lowering the trauma that occurs with tissue injury.

It also inhibits the release of histamine and other inflammatory substances from mast cells. (Mast cells, which are widely distributed throughout the body and are found in highest concentrations in the lining of the respiratory and gastrointestinal tract, the skin, the lining of the joints, and the conjunctiva of the eye, are the usual sites of the allergic and inflammatory responses.)

Because of its antioxidant activity, quercetin also inhibits the formation of leukotrienes, inflammatory compounds that are 1000 times more potent in stimulating inflammatory processes than histamine.

I have found quercetin to be particularly helpful in reducing sensitivity to allergens among my patients. A patient of mine, Janet, suffered from environmental allergies since her teenage years. Her symptoms were particularly bad in the spring, when she would wake up in the morning feeling exhausted and suffering from severe symptoms of nasal congestion, which would continue throughout the day, not clearing until well into the evening.

An artist by profession, she began to paint at night and sleep during the day as a survival strategy. She found all medications to be relatively ineffective in providing adequate symptom relief. However, after beginning a program of natural anti-inflammatory supplements, including quercetin, her symptoms resolved rapidly, and she was able to return to her former work schedule.

Besides environmental allergies, quercetin is also used in the treatment of food allergies, which occur with such common foods as milk, wheat, eggs, soy, strawberries, and peanuts in susceptible people.

Quercetin is effective in the treatment of other inflammatory and allergic conditions including hay fever, allergy, asthma, gout, eczema, arthritis and rheumatoid arthritis, lupus, ulcerative colitis, and Crohn's disease, as well as diabetes and cancer.

It has been successfully used to prevent injury and bruising in athletes and to speed recovery of acutely injured athletes and other performers. Quercetin is also beneficial for the heart, preventing platelet aggregation and promoting relaxation of cardiovascular smooth muscle. It also helps to regulate blood pressure and heart rate. Furthermore, quercetin has been shown to be effective in fighting viral disease and cancer.

Suggested Dosage: Quercetin is not absorbed well by the body unless taken in combination with bromelain, which has been shown to increase its absorption and tissue concentration. Quercetin is available in various strengths; 300 to 600 mg, once or twice a day, is usually effective. Quercetin is well tolerated even in very large quantities. However, it can interfere with estrogen production and reduce menstrual flow. It should be used cautiously by menstruating women.

Curcumin (Turmeric)

Traditional ethnic foods are often flavored with spices that have medicinal properties, which is good reason for regularly including more exotic dishes in your diet. Turmeric, an essential ingredient in curry powder, is a perennial herb of the ginger family and is extensively cultivated in India, China, Indonesia, and other tropical countries. Curcumin is the active medicinal ingredient contained in the thick rhizome of turmeric and gives turmeric its characteristic orange-yellow color.

For thousands of years, curcumin has been used in both Chinese and Indian systems of medicine as an anti-inflammatory agent and for the treatment of numerous health conditions. Modern research corroborates its use as an anti-inflammatory.

A review article on curcumin, published in the *American Journal of Natural Medicine*, summarized several studies done in India that document the usefulness of curcumin as an anti-inflammatory agent.

In one clinical trial, patients with rheumatoid arthritis were given either curcumin (1200 mg per day) or phenylbutazone (300 mg per day), an anti-inflammatory drug known to have serious side effects. The patients were then assessed for the length of time they were able to walk, persistence of morning stiffness, and degree of swelling in the joints. When the results were tabulated, researchers found curcumin to be as beneficial as the drug therapy in reducing symptoms.

In another study, curcumin was also found to be as effective as cortisone, a potent medical anti-inflammatory. This article noted that an added benefit of curcumin is that it does not normally cause side effects, providing a safe alternative to these powerful anti-inflammatory drugs, which can cause gastric irritation and even peptic ulcers in susceptible people.

Curcumin's therapeutic benefits happen through several mechanisms. It reduces inflammation by inhibiting platelet aggregation and leukotriene formation. It also promotes the breakup of blood clots and inhibits the inflammatory response to various stimuli. There is some indication that curcumin has an indirect effect on reducing inflammation through the adrenal gland or its hormones.

The most likely explanation is that it increases the effectiveness of the body's own cortisone, one of the body's major anti-inflammatory hormones. Curcumin may do this by sensitizing or priming cortisone receptor sites, thereby potentiating cortisone's action. It may also act by increasing the half-life of cortisone through reducing its breakdown by the liver.

While the long-term use of prescription cortisone has been associated with serious side effects, including adrenal atrophy, osteoporosis, and diabetes mellitus, curcumin has been found to be as effective as cortisone with no toxicity.

Suggested Dosage: The recommended dosage for curcumin as an anti-inflammatory agent is 400 to 600 mg three times a day. It is often formulated with an equal amount of bromelain to enhance absorption. This combination is best taken on an empty stomach, twenty minutes before meals or between meals. Toxicity reactions have not been reported at standard dosage levels.

Ginger

Ginger is a pungent, spicy herb native to southern Asia. For thousands of years, ginger has been an important herb used in Traditional Chinese Medicine. It is now cultivated throughout the tropics in countries as diverse as Jamaica, India, and China. It is used as a spice in many cuisines and as a flavoring agent for beverages such as ginger ale and in many baked goods.

Ginger is a powerful anti-inflammatory agent. It works by modulating or balancing the prostaglandin pathway. Chemicals in ginger have been found to inhibit inflammatory chemicals like thromboxanes and leukotrienes, which have been linked to conditions like asthma and coronary-artery spasm. On the other hand, these chemicals do not interfere with the production of beneficial anti-inflammatory prostaglandins. As a result, ginger has been found to reduce inflammation, pain, and fever in a variety of conditions. Its effects are similar to medications like aspirin, without the toxic side effects.

Suggested Dosage: Dry, powdered ginger root can be used in dosages of 500 to 1000 mg per day. Tripling or quadrupling this dosage may provide more rapid relief. However, dosages should not be used beyond this level.

Essential Fatty Acids

Essential fatty acids are fats that our body does not produce and that we must therefore obtain through our diet. They consist of two types of special fats: the omega-6 family made up of linoleic acid and the omega-3 family made up of alpha-linolenic acid, EPA (eicosapentaenoic acid), and DHA (docosahexaenoic acid).

While these essential fatty acids supply stored energy in the form of calories, they also perform many other important functions in the body. Essential fatty acids are components of the membrane structure of all cells in the body. They are required for normal development and function of the brain, eyes, inner ear, adrenal glands, and reproductive tract. These essential oils are also necessary for the synthesis of prostaglandins series 1 and 3 hormone-like chemicals that, among other functions, reduce inflammation.

Linoleic acid (omega-6 family) is found in seeds and seed oils. Good sources include flaxseed oil, safflower oil, sunflower oil, and sesame seed oil. Linoleic acid is converted in the body to the anti-inflammatory series-1 prostaglandins.

However, some individuals are unable to synthesize this conversion since their bodies cannot efficiently convert linoleic acid (omega-6 family) to gamma linolenic acid (GLA), an intermediary in the conversion process. Once GLA has been produced, the body can easily continue with the chemical processes needed for the production of series 1 prostaglandin.

To bypass this potential block, individuals can take medicinal seed oils such as evening primrose oil, borage seed oil, and black currant seed oil. These oils contain preformed GLA.

The other common anti-inflammatory essential fatty acids, the omega-3 fatty acids, are found in abundance in fish oil. The best sources are cold-water, high-fat fish such as salmon, tuna, rainbow trout, mackerel, and eel. The only good plant sources of this fatty acid are flaxseeds, soybeans, pumpkin seeds, and walnuts.

In contrast, fats in red meat and poultry skin contain arachidonic acid. Arachidonic acid is converted within the body to the series 2 prostaglandins, which promote inflammation. To manage conditions that involve inflammation, the diet must predominate in fatty acids that convert to the series 1 and series 3 prostaglandins, rather than the fats found in animal foods.

Suggested Dosage: Flaxseed oil can be used in a maximum dosage of 1 to 2 tbsp. of raw oil per day (do not cook with this oil since it is heat sensitive). Fish oil can be taken in dosages of between 2000-3000 mg per day of the omega-3 fatty acids, EPA and DHA.

The therapeutic dosage for borage seed oil is two to four capsules per day, while evening primrose oil requires as many as thirteen capsules a day for maximum therapeutic benefit.

Magnesium

Magnesium and calcium are essential minerals that make up the structure of the bones and also regulate the tone of the nerves and muscles. Calcium is present in beans, turnip greens, tofu, figs, hazelnuts, and blackstrap molasses. It is also present in dairy products, but because of the high incidence of lactose intolerance, may not be as well absorbed as the calcium contained within other foods. Foods that contain magnesium include soybeans, spinach, cashews, pumpkin seeds, and egg yolks.

Since calcium and magnesium have complementary and opposing effects, the objective of treatment is to raise cellular levels of magnesium while lowering levels of calcium. Magnesium helps relax muscles and stabilize mast cells, preventing them from bursting and releasing a flood of histamine, thereby triggering an allergic reaction. In contrast, calcium stimulates mast cells to release histamines.

Magnesium is also particularly useful in the treatment of asthma by reducing inflammation and relaxing the smooth muscle in the lungs. Intravenous magnesium sulfate relaxes the smooth muscle and rapidly opens the bronchial tubes.

Calcium also participates in inflammatory reactions as part of calcium-dependent carrier proteins, which transport proteins to seal off an area and increase inflammation. In individuals with inflammatory conditions, the normal calcium to magnesium ratio of 2:1 can be modified to 1:1 or even 1:2.

Suggested Dosage: At many hospitals, intravenous magnesium sulfate is used, along with prescription drugs, to treat asthmatic attacks. While only a medical professional can administer intravenous magnesium, magnesium supplements taken orally can easily be found in most pharmacies and health food stores and are safe over the long term.

A suggested dosage is 500 to 1000 mg per day. Magnesium does have a laxative effect when used in too high a dosage. If you begin to have loose bowel movements, cut back on the dosage.

Vitamin C

Unlike most animals that produce their own vitamin C, we humans must include it in our diet because our bodies are unable to synthesize it. Because vitamin C is water soluble, it does not accumulate in the body and is rapidly eliminated in urine and through perspiration. Most ingested vitamin C is excreted from the body within three or four hours. If high blood levels of vitamin C are needed, it must be taken at regular intervals throughout the day. In addition, its potency can be lost through exposure to light, heat, and air.

Vitamin C reduces inflammation by decreasing histamine levels in the blood. In an allergic response, histamine levels tend to rise. In a study published in the *Journal of Nutrition*, oral supplementation of vitamin C at 1 g per day for three days in eleven volunteers reduced blood histamine levels in every case.

This same paper noted that in evaluating 437 human blood samples, when plasma vitamin C levels fell below 1 mg/100 ml, whole blood histamine levels increased exponentially as the ascorbic-acid level decreased. Besides reducing histamines, vitamin C is also needed for the synthesis of adrenal cortico-steroids, our body's own anti-inflammatory agents.

Vitamin C can have a laxative effect, enabling the patient to pass food through the intestinal tract more efficiently and completely. This too can be helpful in treating allergies. When a person is constipated, fecal material remains in the intestine long enough for toxins to be reabsorbed from the bowel back into the bloodstream. These reabsorbed toxins can exacerbate allergies.

When vitamin C is combined with digestive enzymes and hesperidin (a bioflavonoid commonly found in citrus peel), it can also be used successfully to speed recovery time in sports injuries.

Suggested Dosage: Since vitamin C has a laxative effect, initial doses should be low, such as 500 to 1000 mg, one to three times a day. Higher doses of vitamin C can be used safely, and people with inflammatory conditions may use as much as 5,000 to 10,000 mg of vitamin C as a total dosage. While high doses of vitamin C can be very helpful, not everyone can tolerate this because of bowel sensitivity and its laxative effect.

Start with 1 to 3 g per day, increasing your intake to bowel tolerance. If your stools become loose, drop to a level that permits a normal bowel movement. To accelerate recovery from injuries, 750 mg of citrus bioflavonoids, one to two capsules per day, can be used along with vitamin C.

Many people who are overly acidic often experience stomach or intestinal-tract discomfort when using vitamin C in the form of ascorbic acid. In such cases, be sure to use a buffered form of vitamin C. It can be buffered by the addition of alkaline minerals such as sodium, calcium, potassium, or magnesium and still maintain its active properties. Buffered vitamin C also reduces the laxative and gastric-irritant effects of ascorbic acid, which is helpful for people with poor bowel tolerance of this very important nutrient.

11

Other Beneficial Nutrients and Good Habits to Promote Healthy Digestive Function

If you have chronic digestive complaints such as gas, bloating, abdominal discomfort, or poor bowel function, usually more than simply weak pancreatic function is involved.

Millions of people also suffer from such common conditions as intestinal food allergies, irritable-bowel syndrome, colitis, and gastritis. These conditions become particularly common after midlife and reflect the weakening and diminished functional capability of the digestive organs in general.

In such cases, a nutritional program to support the function of the digestive tract may be helpful. I have included a number of substances in this section that can be helpful in supporting, and even restoring, better digestive function, as well as two good habits that you should try to develop to help your body's digestive process.

Hydrochloric Acid

Hydrochloric acid (HCl) is produced by the parietal cells of the stomach, primarily to begin the task of breaking down proteins so that they can be properly digested. HCl is needed to lower the pH of the stomach. In fact, stomach acid is so strong that it is as much as 100,000 to nearly 1,000,000 times more acidic than water.

HCl also activates the proteolytic enzyme pepsin found in the stomach. A lack of either or both will interfere with normal digestion. HCl also makes nutrients like calcium, iron, and vitamin B12 more absorbable and helps to suppress the growth of disease-causing bacteria in the stomach.

As we age, some individuals may produce less HCl. Several research studies have found reduced HCl production in more than half of volunteers examined over the age of sixty. Although other studies contradict these findings, you should be aware that a normal physiological decline in stomach acid can occur in certain individuals. This condition should be properly diagnosed and treated with HCl supplementation. Emotional stress, poor diet, and exposure to toxins can also impair our ability to produce HCl.

Low gastric acidity is associated with many diseases, including asthma, rheumatoid arthritis, and gallbladder disease. In addition, low gastric acidity may also contribute to the overgrowth of bacteria in the small bowel. Common symptoms of low gastric acidity are bloating, belching, flatulence immediately after eating, diarrhea, constipation, food allergies, and nausea after taking supplements.

Individuals who are overly acidic may find that the use of hydrochloric acid worsens digestive symptoms such as heartburn and abdominal discomfort. If this applies to you, be sure to read the label of any digestive aid before buying it to make sure that it does not contain hydrochloric acid. If you have sufficient or even too much acid production, HCl may aggravate your symptoms, giving you heartburn, and should be discontinued immediately.

Suggested Dosage: Begin by taking one tablet or capsule containing 10 grains (600 mg) of hydrochloric acid at your next meal. If well tolerated, take one tablet or capsule at the next meal and increase the dosage by one tablet or capsule at every subsequent meal. (That is, one at the next meal, two at the meal after that, then three at the next meal.) Continue to increase the dose until you reach seven tablets or until you feel a warmth in your stomach, whichever occurs first.

After you have found the largest dose that you can take at mealtime without feeling any warmth, maintain that dose at all meals of similar size. You will need to take less at smaller meals, however.

When taking a number of tablets or capsules, you should take them throughout the meal. It is very important not to take HCl on an empty stomach, and HCl is contraindicated in persons with peptic-ulcer disease. Because HCl can irritate sensitive tissue and can be corrosive to teeth, capsules should not be emptied into food or dissolved in beverages.

Cider Vinegar

Many people have found that taking 1 to 2 tbsp per day of cider vinegar will have similar effects as supplementing with hydrochloric acid, with fewer negative side effects. Be sure to use raw, unpasteurized, unfiltered cider vinegar made from organic apples. For those whose stomach acid production is compromised, the cider vinegar seems to be less harsh to the stomach lining. The primary acid in cider vinegar is malic acid. Malate is a component of the Kreb's cycle, a series of chemical reactions involved in the conversion of food to energy.

Overly acidic individuals should be conservative in their use of HCl or cider vinegar because it will add to their acid load and they will feel discomfort after taking it. Use these supplements with great caution, or not at all, if you have conditions related to over acidity. However, if you feel you may be deficient in stomach acid, you can try cider vinegar instead of beginning with commercial preparations of HCl.

Lactobacilli and Bifidobacteria

Friendly bacteria like lactobacilli and bifidobacteria normally colonize the intestinal tract. These bacteria have many beneficial effects on digestion. Because they aid in the production of essential B vitamins as well as acetic and lactic acids, they prevent colonization of the colon by harmful bacteria and yeast.

However, overconsumption of alcohol or sugar, a high-fat diet, and the use of antibiotics can reduce the population of lactobacilli and predispose the body to an overgrowth of harmful bacteria and fungi. Pathogenic organisms like candida may flourish in this environment.

I have worked with numerous patients who have been given antibiotics to treat such common health conditions as bronchitis and the flu and have consequently developed candida. The vaginal itching, burning, and discharge due to overgrowth of candida in the vagina and intestines then has to be treated as a separate infection.

To insure healthy intestinal flora, I recommend taking lactobacilli supplements on a regular basis. For maximum effectiveness, take these on an empty stomach, in the morning and one hour before meals.

Various cultures are available as powders, capsules, tablets, and liquids, measured by the amount of viable bacteria per dosage.

For those people who can tolerate dairy products, soured milk products such as buttermilk, yogurt, acidophilus milk, and kefir can also be used to help restore the levels of friendly bacteria. There are also nondairy acidophilus products, such as soy yogurt, for people who are allergic to dairy foods.

Fiber

Dietary fiber can improve the function and absorptive capacity of the intestinal tract. Insoluble fibers such as cellulose and hemicellulose are found in fruits, vegetables, nuts, and beans. Soluble fibers like pectins, gums, and mucilages are found in oatmeal, oat bran, sesame seeds, and dried beans. Because the refining process has removed most of the natural fiber from our foods, the average American's diet is grossly lacking in fiber.

Fiber helps prevent constipation, colon cancer, and many other intestinal disorders. (More than 85,000 cases of colon cancer are diagnosed each year.) Once ingested, fiber undergoes bacterial fermentation in the colon. This process produces butyrate, the main energy source for colonic epithelial cells, which are needed for a healthy, cancer-free colon.

This effect was verified in a study published in the *Scandinavian Journal of Gastroenterology*. Researchers followed the health of twenty patients who had undergone surgical treatment for colon cancer. The volunteers were given fiber in the form of psyllium seeds. After one month of supplementation, fecal concentration of butyrate increased by 47 percent.

Fiber may also help to decrease the tendency toward over acidity in the intestinal tract by reducing inflammation. This occurs because fiber improves the transit time of food as it moves through the intestinal tract; it also promotes the growth of beneficial intestinal flora. These flora are less acidifying and irritating to the intestines than are the less healthy flora that thrive when people eat low-fiber, high-fat, high-sugar diets.

High-energy activities and peak performance require proper bowel function, so that food moves quickly through the intestines and toxic waste products are eliminated. To increase your fiber intake, include in your meals whole-grain cereals and flours, brown rice, all kinds of bran, fruits such as apricots, dried prunes, and apples (unless you tend to be overly acidic), nuts, seeds, beans, lentils, peas, and vegetables. Several of these foods should be included in every meal. Moreover, when you eat apples and potatoes, enjoy them with their skins.

Suggested Dosage: If you supplement your diet with fiber, start with small amounts and gradually increase your intake. Fiber like oat bran and psyllium should be used to a maximum dosage of 1 to 2 tbsp. per day. This should be taken mixed with 8 to 12 oz. of water and swallowed immediately after stirring, since psyllium can become gel-like in texture.

Those suffering from Crohn's disease (an inflammatory condition of the small intestine that can cause abdominal pain, cramping, and change in bowel habits) should avoid supplemental fiber and only consume fiber in foods. Soluble fiber like guar gum and pectin (derived from apples and grapefruit) can be taken in the same manner.

Combine ½ tsp. guar gum and 500 mg of pectin and add this mixture to 8 to 12 oz. of water. Stir and drink immediately. Use one to three times a day.

Herbs

Many herbs and spices are time-honored digestive aids. My patients often use herbal teas as a healthy and satisfying alternative to acidic coffee. I also have many patients who drink coffee in the morning for a quick energy boost.

However, this boost is only temporary; after an hour or two, most individuals have difficulty staying alert enough to focus on work and meet deadlines without drinking additional coffee.

Ginger and peppermint teas are made from mildly stimulating herbs and can produce more subtle but sustained increases in energy. Many herbs can be used as a delicious morning beverage and have beneficial effects on both mental alertness and digestive function without causing the side effects and addiction of caffeine.

Peppermint tea also helps alleviate gas by acting as a stomach sedative and powerful antispasmodic. Chamomile tea soothes the digestive tract and also acts as a natural antispasmodic, reducing pain and discomfort.

Fennel disperses gas and dispels bloating. (For this purpose, a traditional Indian curry dinner ends with a bowl of fennel.) Finally, licorice, the sweet-tasting herb used to flavor candy, has been found to be quite effective in the treatment of peptic ulcers. Research studies have shown that licorice strengthens the protective lining of the intestinal tract and helps to prevent ulcer formation.

Water

For optimal digestive health and hydration of body tissues, drink eight to ten glasses of water a day. This should be done apart from liquid taken with meals. Fluids stimulate the production of saliva, bile, and gastric, pancreatic, and intestinal juices. The water should be drunk at room temperature.

Non-chlorinated spring or filtered water is best. There is ongoing controversy over whether taking fluids with meals dilutes digestive enzymes or stimulates their production. I recommend reducing fluid intake with meals and drinking most of your water between meals.

Two Good Habits

You can also improve your digestive function by developing two simple habits that will make an important difference in your health: (1) chew your food thoroughly, and (2) eat your last meal of the day in the early evening.

Chew Your Food Thoroughly

This maternal advice still holds true. The longer you chew your food, the longer the enzymes in your mouth have to begin the work of digestion. The starch-digesting enzyme ptyalin helps to break up starches even before they are swallowed.

Chewing is critical for digestion of all foods, because enzymes only act on the surface area of food particles. The more time you spend chewing your food, the more surface area of food will be exposed to enzymes, leading to better digestion.

Raw fruits and vegetables, although good sources of living enzymes, need to be chewed very thoroughly because they contain cellulose membranes that are indigestible must be broken before nutrients can be released and the food digested.

Chewing triggers the body's production of digestive enzymes and stimulates the secretion of pancreatic fluids, intestinal juices, and bile (an emulsifying agent produced by the liver that is essential for the digestion of fats). Gulping down a sandwich in ten minutes so that you can use the rest of your lunch hour for catching up on work does not serve your health in the long run.

Eat Your Last Meal of the Day in the Early Evening

Eating late at night puts stress on the organs in the digestive system. It is preferable to complete your final meal of the day by 7:00 p.m. It is also important to eat in a relaxed state and not to try to negotiate a major deal over dinner. To maintain the health and stamina you need to be successful in business or any creative endeavor, you need to make mealtime a peaceful and relaxing experience.

Summary of Treatment Options for Restoring Your Digestive Enzymes

Diet

Choose enzyme-rich foods

Avoid foods that stress the pancreas

Drink blenderized drinks, if indicated

Eat pureed foods, if indicated

Supplemental digestive enzymes

Plant-based digestive enzymes

Bromelain

Papain

Pancreatic enzymes derived from animal sources

Other natural anti-inflammatory agents

MSM (methylsulfonylmethane)

Colloidal silver

Colostrum

Alkalinizing agents

Quercetin

Curcumin (turmeric)

Ginger

Essential fatty acids

Magnesium and calcium

Vitamin C

Digestive aids

Hydrochloric acid
Cider vinegar
Lactobacilli and bifidobacteria
Fiber
Culinary herbs
Water

About Susan Richards, M.D.

Dr. Susan Richards is one of the foremost authorities in the fields of family medicine and alternative medicine. Dr. Richards has successfully treated many thousands of patients emphasizing alternative health and integrative medicine in her clinical practice. Her mission is to provide her patients with safe and effective alternative therapies to greatly enhance their health and well-being.

A graduate of Northwestern University Feinberg School of Medicine, she has served on the clinical faculty of Stanford University School of Medicine and taught in their Division of Family and Community Medicine.

Her Facebook page, Dr. Susan's Healthy Living, has over one million followers. She is also an ordained minister and her ministry receives over a million prayer requests for healing each year.

Notes

Notes

Notes

www.ingramcontent.com/pod-product-compliance
Lightning Source LLC
Chambersburg PA
CBHW070907290526
45795CB00001B/235